Our Commitment

At Johnson & Johnson, we believe that nurses are the backbone of health systems, who bring innovation, expertise and resourcefulness to profoundly improve patient care and health outcomes around the world.

Today, we are proud to continue our 120-year commitment to advocating for and supporting the nursing profession by elevating the profile of nurses as innovative leaders and empowering them to deliver at their full potential.

Because nurses change lives, and that changes everything.

Learn more at nursing.jnj.com.

Johnson & Johnson

THE REBEL NURSE HANDBOOK

Rebecca Love, MSN, BS, RN, FIEL
President, Society of Nurse Scientists, Innovators, Entrepreneurs, and Leaders (SONSIEL)

Rebecca Love is a nurse entrepreneur, inventor, author, Tedx speaker, the first nurse featured on Ted.com, and part of the inaugural nursing panel featured at SXSW 2018. Love was the first Director of Nurse Innovation and Entrepreneurship in the United States at Northeastern School of Nursing—a founding initiative designed to empower nurses as innovators and entrepreneurs. There she founded the Nurse Hackathon; the movement has led to transformational change in the nursing profession.

Rebecca is an experienced nurse entrepreneur, founding HireNurses.com in 2013 (acquired in 2018), and currently serves as the President of SONSIEL. In early 2019, Rebecca, along with a group of leading nurses in the world, founded SONSIEL: The Society of Nurse Scientists, Innovators, Entrepreneurs, and Leaders. Love is passionate about empowering nurses and creating communities to help nurses innovate, create, and collaborate to start businesses and inventions to transform healthcare.

Rebecca holds an MS in Nursing from Northeastern University and a BA in International Relations/Spanish from Boston University; she is currently a faculty member at Norwich University and sits on the board of NextGen Ventures and the Host Committee for the Massachusetts American Civil Liberties Union (ACLU). She currently lives in Marblehead, Massachusetts, with her husband and three children.

Nancy Hanrahan, PhD, RN, FAAN

Nancy Hanrahan is an experienced professor and leader with a joy for creating opportunities for nurses and spreading the often-unknown value of nurses for safe, healing healthcare environments. Her skills include the following areas: education development, behavioral health, research of mental health services, healthcare innovation and entrepreneurship, public health, public speaking, and transformational leadership. Her PhD focused on mental health service research from Boston College and her postdoctoral study was at the University of Pennsylvania at the Center for Health Outcomes and Policy Research. Dr. Hanrahan leads the Nurse Innovation and Entrepreneurship Institute at University of Massachusetts at Boston. This program empowers nurses to lead research and innovation that transform health systems using big data, to redesign the healthcare experience of patients and families, and to engage patients in meaningful health behavior change. Her work has been widely published and has received national and international awards for development of innovative interventions. She is cofounder of the Society of Nurse Scientists, Innovators, Entrepreneurs, and Leaders (www.sonsiel.com) and principal/cofounder of Nurse Approved, LLC (www.nurseapproved.health).

Mary Lou Ackerman, MBA, BScN
Vice President, Innovation and Digital Health

Mary Lou Ackerman is vice president of Innovation and Digital Health with SE Health. Ms. Ackerman is a founding member of the Society of Nurse Scientists, Innovators, Entrepreneurs, and Leaders (SONSIEL) and an active member of Canada's Health Informatics Executive Forum (CHIEF) with Digital Health Canada. Her background is extensive—she has led the development and implementation of many business transformation projects, innovations, and partnerships. She joined Saint Elizabeth in 1987 as a visiting nurse, and she has augmented her clinical background with a graduate business degree and significant experience with health informatics, innovation, and digital health. Ms. Ackerman has a passion for community healthcare, combined with a desire to advance care, creating innovative service models supported by digital health technologies, to create a future that will provide a personalized, accessible, meaningful health experience for individuals, their families, and the service providers who support them.

Amy Rose Taylor, AGNP-BC, BSN, RN
Clinical Services Manager and Podcast Host, UnitedHealth Group Pennsylvania

Amy Rose Taylor earned a degree in English from the University of Hawaii–Manoa and her nursing degrees from Columbia University. While at Columbia, she was selected as a Jonas Scholar, a Columbia Nurse Leader, and a Columbia-Macy Interprofessional Scholar, and was the research assistant to Dean Emeritus Mary O. Mundinger. She was selected as the Health Policy Fellow for the American Association of Nurse Practitioners in Washington, DC. Recently, she was honored as an inaugural Leadership Academy Member for the Geriatric Advanced Practice Nurse Association and is proud to be a founding member of SONSIEL. She currently works as a clinical services manager for UnitedHealth Group and is the host of Clinician Commons Live Podcast, the official podcast for UnitedHealth Group. She enjoys podcasting, as it reminds her of her youth as an international journalist, having interviewed guests as varied as Michael Jackson to Nancy Reagan. She currently lives in New York with her five children and her supportive husband, Joe.

Elizabeth Toner, MJ, MSN, RN

Beth Toner is senior communications officer at the Robert Wood Johnson Foundation. She has more than 28 years of experience in marketing and corporate communications; she is also a registered nurse with clinical experience in long-term care and community health settings.

Toner joined the Foundation in 2012 from The Hartford, where she was director of marketing initiatives for the Advanced Markets Group. Prior to her work with The Hartford, Toner was a senior web content developer for the Children's Hospital of Philadelphia. She has also served as a multimedia communications specialist for the University of Pennsylvania Health System and a public relations coordinator for Harleysville Insurance.

Toner holds an associate of applied science in nursing degree from Delaware County Community College, a bachelor's degree in communications from Messiah College, a master of journalism degree from Temple University, and a master of science in nursing from Eastern Mennonite University.

Faith Ann Lawlor, RN
Operations, Society of Nurse Scientists, Innovators, Entrepreneurs, and Leaders (SONSIEL)

Ms. Lawlor executes events, oversees membership services, and implements technology, financial, and marketing solutions for SONSIEL. Faith is an experienced leader, with an analytical and strategic mind, and proven track record in delivering results in a high-stakes environment. Ms. Lawlor has extensive knowledge in business, nursing, and healthcare.

THE REBEL NURSE HANDBOOK

Inspirational Stories by Shift Disruptors

Rebecca Love, MSN, BS, RN, FIEL

Nancy Hanrahan, PhD, RN, FAAN

Mary Lou Ackerman, MBA, BScN

Faith Ann Lawlor, RN

Amy Rose Taylor, AGNP-BC, BSN, RN

Elizabeth Toner, MJ, MSN, RN

SPRINGER PUBLISHING COMPANY

Springer Publishing Company, LLC
11 West 42nd Street, New York, NY 10036
www.springerpub.com
connect.springerpub.com

Acquisitions Editor: Elizabeth Nieginski
Editor: Hannah M. Hicks
Compositor: diacriTech

ISBN: 978-0-8261-5143-8
ebook ISBN: 978-0-8261-5144-5
DOI: 10.1891/9780826151445

20 21 22 23 / 5 4 3 2 1

The author and the publisher of this Work have made every effort to use sources believed to be reliable to provide information that is accurate and compatible with the standards generally accepted at the time of publication. The author and publisher shall not be liable for any special, consequential, or exemplary damages resulting, in whole or in part, from the readers' use of, or reliance on, the information contained in this book. The publisher has no responsibility for the persistence or accuracy of URLs for external or third-party Internet websites referred to in this publication and does not guarantee that any content on such websites is, or will remain, accurate or appropriate.

The names of people mentioned in this book have been used with permission. Otherwise, information has been changed to protect identities.

Library of Congress Cataloging-in-Publication Data
Library of Congress Control Number: 2019919463

Rebecca Love: https://orcid.org/0000-0002-8039-4163
Nancy Hanrahan: https://orcid.org/0000-0003-2856-8557
Mary Lou Ackerman: https://orcid.org/0000-0001-9072-6064
Faith Ann Lawlor: https://orcid.org/0000-0002-8039-4163
Amy Rose Taylor: https://orcid.org/0000-0002-8039-4163
Elizabeth Toner: https://orcid.org/0000-0002-5663-0429

Publisher's Note: New and used products purchased from third-party sellers are not guaranteed for quality, authenticity, or access to any included digital components.

Printed in the United States of America.

To all the resilient, inspiring, and myth-busting nurses destined to disrupt the future of nursing. Thank you for being a rebel with a cause.

Contents

Contributors

Mary Lou Ackerman, MBA, BScN, Vice President Innovation and Digital Health, SE Health, Toronto, Ontario, Canada

Nancy M. Albert, PhD, CCNS, CHFN, CCRN, NE-BC, FAHA, FCCM, FHFSA, FAAN, Associate Chief Nursing Officer, Research and Innovation-Nursing Institute, Clinical Nurse Specialist, Heart Failure, Kaufman Center for Heart Failure, Heart and Vascular Institute, Cleveland Clinic, Cleveland, Ohio

Shawna Butler, DNP, JD, RN, CPHRM, Patient Safety Specialist/Research Nurse Coordinator/Nurse, Massachusetts General Hospital, Boston, Massachusetts, and Nursing Faculty, University of Massachusetts, Boston, Massachusetts

Keith Carlson, BSN, RN, NC-BC, Nurse Career Coach, Podcaster, Writer, Motivational Speaker, Nurse Keith Coaching, Santa Fe, New Mexico

Bonnie Clipper, DNP, RN, MA, MBA, CENP, FACHE, Chief Clinical Officer, Wambi, Austin, Texas

Paul E. Coyne, DNP, MBA, MS, RN, APRN, AGPCNP-BC, President and Cofounder, Inspiren, New York, New York, and Assistant Vice President, Clinical Practice & Chief Nursing Informatics Officer, Hospital for Special Surgery, New York, New York

Sheila Davis, DNP, ANP-BC, FAAN, Chief Executive Officer, Partners in Health, Boston, Massachusetts

Stephan Davis, DNP, MHSA, NEA-BC, CENP, CNE, FACHE, FIEL, Founder and Principal, Illuminant, and Clinical Assistant Professor, Georgia State University, Atlanta, Georgia

Margaret A. Fitzgerald, DNP, FNP-BC, NP-C, FAANP, CSP, FAAN, DCC, FNAP, President, Fitzgerald Health Education Associates, North Andover, Massachusetts, Clinical Practice, Family Nurse Practitioner, Greater Lawrence, Massachusetts, Family Health Center, Lawrence, Massachusetts, Adjunct Associate Professor, Frances Payne Bolton School of Nursing, Case Western Reserve University, Cleveland, Ohio

Janie Harvey Garner, RN, Founder of Show Me Your Stethoscope, LLC, Founder of the SMYS Foundation, Hillsboro, Missouri

Debbie Gregory, DNP, RN, Coeditor, HERD Journal, Adjunct Professor, Vanderbilt University School of Nursing, Adjunct Professor, Clemson University School of Nursing, Senior Clinical Consultant, Smith, Seckman, Reid, Inc., Nashville, Tennessee

Shailadi Gupta, BScN, RN, Kindshell Global CEO and Founder

Nancy Hanrahan, PhD, RN, FAAN, Professor, University of Massachusetts, Boston, and Executive Director, Innovation and Entrepreneurship, Boston, Massachusetts

Noah Hendler, MSN, MPS, RN, APRN, FNP-C, Nurse Practitioner, Consultant, Investor, Care Architect, LLC, Fairfield, Connecticut

Andrea Jaramillo, BSN, RN, Labor & Delivery Staff Nurse, Boston Medical Center, Boston, Massachusetts

Jalil Johnson, PhD, MS, APRN, ANP-BC, Nurse Activist, CEO SMYS Foundation, Northampton, Massachusetts

Joyce M. Knestrick, PhD, RN, FNP-BC, FAANP, Immediate Past President, American Association of Nurse Practitioners, Pittsburgh, Pennsylvania, and Visiting Professor, George Washington University, Washington, DC

Paul Kuehnert, DNP, RN, FAAN, Associate Vice President-Program, Robert Wood Johnson Foundation, Princeton, New Jersey, Affiliate Professor of Nursing, University of Washington, Seattle, Washington

Kelly Larrabee-Robke, MBA, MS, BSN, RN, Vice President, Clinical Thought Leadership, BD Medical Affairs, San Diego, California

Michael Lawler, MSN, BS, RN, FNP-BC, EMBA, MGCP, Founder & Chief Operations Operator of Biilt Contracting Group, Founder & CEO, Kynamics Consulting Partners, MedOptions Family Nurse Practitioner

Faith Ann Lawlor, RN, Operations, Society of Nurse Scientists, Innovators, Entrepreneurs, and Leaders (SONSIEL), Boston, Massachusetts

Marion Leary, MSN, MPH, RN, Director of Innovation, School of Nursing, University of Pennsylvania, Philadelphia, Pennsylvania

Nicole Lincoln, MS, RN, FNP-BC, CCNS, CCRN, Senior Manager of Nursing Innovations, Boston Medical Center, Boston, Massachusetts

Rebecca Love, MSN, BS, RN, FIEL, Cofounder and President of Society of Nurse Scientists, Innovators, Entrepreneurs, and Leaders (SONSIEL), Boston, Massachusetts

Rhonda Manns, MBA, BSN, RN, Registered Nurse Case Manager, Optum/UnitedHealthcare, Atlanta, Georgia

Bobbi Martin, MSN, RN, President and CEO, Global Nurse Network, Indian Rocks Beach, Florida

Brittany Molkenthin, BSN, RN, CPN, CEO, Lactation Innovations LLC, Canterbury, Connecticut

Martie Moore, MAOM, RN, CPHQ, Chief Nursing Officer, Medline Industries, Inc., Chicago, Illinois

Richard Moore, PhD, DProf(c), MBA, MSc (Cardiology), BSc (Hons), RN, RNT, DMS, FIMGT, FHEA, FESC, FIEL, FRSPH, JP, School of Medicine & School of International Finance & Management, Pyongyang University of Science & Technology, Pyongyang, North Korea, Indigenous Learning Advisor, Indigenous Education & Research Centre, James Cook University, Cairns, Australia

Hiyam M. Nadel, RN, MBA, CGC, Director, The Center of Innovations in Care Delivery, Massachusetts General Hospital, Boston, Massachusetts

Nancy Nager, MSN, RN, President/CEO, Specialized Healthcare Services, Needham, Massachusetts

Christine M. O'Brien, DNP, MSHI, RN-BC, FIEL, Associate Director of Clinical Informatics, Tufts Medical Center, Boston, Massachusetts

Chinelo Ofoma, MSN, RN, CPNP-PC, FIEL, Pediatric Nurse Practitioner, Founder of Nurse On Purpose | Challenging Media Stereotypes of Nursing

Joan Gurvis Shields, MSN, RN, BCC, Senior Faculty/Leadership Solutions Partner, Center for Creative Leadership, Colorado Springs, Colorado

Bongi Sibanda, DNPc, MSc, ANP, FHEA, RN, Advanced Practice Nurse Consultant/ Educator, Doctoral Candidate, Queen's University Belfast, Belfast, United Kingdom

Veronica Southerland, DNP(s), APRN, FNP-BC, BSW, Family Nurse Practitioner, Advanced Practice Care Clinic, Charlotte, North Carolina

Amy Rose Taylor, AGNP-BC, BSN, RN, Clinical Services Manager, Optum at Home, UnitedHealth Group, Pennsylvania

Elizabeth Toner, MJ, MSN, RN, Senior Communications Officer, Robert Wood Johnson Foundation, Princeton, New Jersey

Debbie Toomey, RN, CIPP, Speaker–Author–Consultant, Founder, President, Ultimate Healing Journey, LLC, Quincy, Massachusetts

Joanna Seltzer Uribe, MSN, RN, EdD, Director of Strategic Design Hourglass Education Technology Solutions, Phoenix, Arizona, Johnson & Johnson Nurse Innovation Fellow 2020–2021

Jennifer Wallace, MSN, RN, Assistant Professor, Family Focused Nursing, Lawrence Memorial Regis College, Medford, Massachusetts

Brian Weirich, DHA, MHA, BSN, CENP, Chief Nurse Executive/Founder, West Lafayette, Indiana

Kevin Whitney, DNP, RN, NEA-BC, Senior Vice President of Patient Care Services and Chief Nursing Officer, Newton-Wellesley Hospital, Newton, Massachusetts

Wendy Wright, DNP, ANP-BC, FNP-BC, FAANP, FAAN, FNAP, Adult and Family Nurse Practitioner, Owner, Wright & Associates Family Healthcare @ Amherst and @ Concord, New Hampshire, Adjunct Faculty, Fay W. Whitney School of Nursing, University of Wyoming, Laramie, Wyoming

Foreword

I often say, "If you are not at the table, then you are on the menu," and it's time that nurses take a seat at the table. Nursing is often absent from the majority of leadership tables of healthcare systems, health plans, and life science/medical device organizations. However, because nursing represents the largest percentage of the healthcare professional workforce, this needs to change. The current nurses need to claim their seats at the table, even bring their own chair, especially when an invitation is not extended.

My own career in nursing is the story of pioneering a different path than the typical nursing career. I worked at the bedside as a neonatal ICU and pediatric nurse for only a few years before I realized that there was a world in healthcare that I wanted to explore. My curiosity in technology from patient monitoring to big data (before "big data" was cool!) drove me to explore outside my comfort zone and seek opportunity and take risks in new roles. As I reflect back on my career, I realize that when I started out as a bedside nurse, I never imagined a career in healthcare and technology and now as the Chief Nursing Officer of Microsoft. But it was taking the road less traveled that led me to the most challenging career in healthcare and technology, and I encourage all of you to do the same and find what you are passionate about and what intellectually sparks your curiosity.

As you read the stories ahead of the incredible, "rock star," "rebel" nurses, each of whom have challenged the status quo and chosen the road less traveled, remember that each journey has its own period of self-doubt, fear of failure, and uncertainty of success—but they persevered. I believe that success comes from an inner belief and confidence that one can make the world a better place—for patients, fellow nurses, and beyond. We hope that these stories will inspire you to believe in yourself and aim a little higher each day.

Go claim your seat.

Molly K. McCarthy, MBA, BSN, RN-BC
National Director, U. S. Provider Industry and Chief Nursing Officer
Microsoft U. S. Health and Life Sciences
Chevy Chase, Maryland

Preface

This book was inspired by you: the nurse unicorn looking for a tribe; the nurse needing inspiration to achieve greater heights; the nurse or future nurse who is not okay with the status quo. It was written with the primary purpose of giving you the opportunity to be inspired by the stories of others.

Each contributor is a Founding Member or Fellow of the Society of Nurse Scientists, Innovators, Entrepreneurs, and Leaders (SONSIEL). Many of these nurses embodied the essence of the *Rebel Nurse* before it was something *chic* to talk about.

This is a compilation of over 40 diverse nurse leaders, innovators, and entrepreneurs, each possessing the same mentality—to change the face of healthcare by thinking outside the norm and moving past traditions. These nurses have lent their stories, their reputations, and their journeys, so that you will now know that others have been through the discomfort you may be experiencing in order to disrupt the status quo.

Through months of collaborative brainstorming, and tweaking and re-tweaking personal stories, we have taken years of experience, thousands of hours of failure and rejection, hundreds of moments of uncertainty, and immeasurable amounts of life-altering situations, to design a book that will give you a snapshot of inspiration, resources, and methodologies to enhance your own toolkit on this *Rebel Nurse* journey.

Each story holds its own special place within chapters designed to carry a common theme between storytellers, as it maps out these nurses' paths into where they find themselves today.

Chapter 1, Shift Disruptors: Stories of Nurses Recognizing Their Unique Role in Healthcare, shares stories of nurses who encountered nursing from both traditional and nontraditional backgrounds, but with a unique twist. Many of these stories may be relevant for the early-career nurses, those who are still finding their own path, as well as those at the cusp of a pivot in their nursing journey. Chapter 2, Overcoming the Odds: Pioneer Nurses Blazing Trails Around the World, shares the unique journeys of nurses who have had to literally overcome major difficulties, challenges, and obstacles within their personal and professional lives. The common theme of these nurses is their incredible display of resilience and strength to create a brand new path for themselves, and in their identity as nurses. Chapter 3, Transforming Your Passion: Innovatively Adaptive Nurses Working Across Multiple Sectors, highlights nurses who have taken their unique passion, vision, or dream—some in the middle season of their careers—both within nursing and beyond, and adapted it to redefine nursing altogether. Some have started businesses, others ventured into the tech world, and some have even integrated nursing with interior design, but they all have uniquely interwoven nursing in a way that surpasses the traditional definition of nursing to impact healthcare in a special way. Chapter 4, The Price of Compassion: Soulful Stories of the Humanity of Nursing, gives a very deep and personal look into the emotional journeys of *rebel nurses*; from "soul drought" to happiness, these nurses demonstrate the (many times) heart-wrenching side of nursing that makes it both a science and an art. Chapter 5, Sharing Their Story: Words of Wisdom by Rebel Nurses Who Disrupted the Status Quo, is a gift from the seasoned nurses of our times. Some of these nurses have just about "seen it all," and are now using their experiences to provide wisdom to the future generations of nursing. And finally, Chapter 6, Rebel Nurses at the Crossroads: Innovative Methodologies, Reflections, and Resources to Guide the Future of Nursing, is a theoretical and practical forecast into nursing and healthcare. It outlines detailed methodologies on innovation and gives a powerful charge into the future of nursing. At the end of each chapter, you will also find "progress notes," or summary points of the major takeaways of each contributing *Rebel Nurse*.

All of these nurses have also provided additional resources to guide you along the way, as each nurse has strategically lined their story with words of wisdom, personal resources, and inspiration that will hopefully continue to propel you forward toward your own mark in history. And, as a bonus, you will also find a variety of publications and authored works by SONSIEL members to fill your bookshelf with the next set of dynamic resources.

As we send you forward into the lives of these amazing nurses, we imagine each of you have had your own moments of resilience, transformation, innovation, courage, and all-around multifaceted character, to revolutionize the way care has been delivered in your sphere of influence. And these inspirational stories will allow you to find a bit of encouragement, motivation, and wisdom, as you see history rewriting itself, with your own story as another strategic piece to the puzzle.

So, our (metaphorical) caps off to you, *Rebel Nurse*. Destined to be in business, tech, or the start-up world? Looking to be innovative in healthcare delivery, in collaboration with a non-traditional platform? If you are the nurse who wants to truly influence the healthcare scene in a way that defines the future of nursing, all of these stories are for you, and we are rooting you on! Thank you for allowing us to share our stories; we hope that you will continue to do the same for others around you.

Sincerely,

Rebecca, Nancy, Amy Rose, Faith, Mary Lou, and Beth
on behalf of SONSIEL (and the *Rebel Nurses* of our time)

Acknowledgments

Coalescing, synthesizing, and streamlining a book of the very personal stories of over 40 different people, let alone rebel nurses, is not an easy task. But the opportunity to share our stories to inspire your own is a truly humbling (and rewarding) honor.

So, to every person who has played a role in crafting this collaborative work, as well as who have been by our side every step of the way, thank you. We would like to especially thank:

Our editor at Springer Publishing Company, Hannah Hicks, whose diligence, patience, expertise, and guidance helped us turn this into a quality work

The entire Springer Publishing Company team, especially Elizabeth Nieginski, who believed in the mission and vision behind this book

All the rebel nurses who paved the way throughout history, those who stepped in and solved the problems they saw without asking for permission, and who use their courage to continue to find the heart of their work despite many obstacles

Our families, who support these crazy dreams and wild pursuits

. . . and the woman who, if she hadn't been a rebel, we would never exist . . . Florence Nightingale

To all the authors daring enough to share their personal stories with the world.

Thank you!

Introduction

Try. Fail. Pivot. Try Again.
The Path to Success.

REBECCA LOVE, MSN, BS, RN, FIEL

> *"WERE THERE NONE WHO WERE DISCONTENTED, THE WORLD*
> *WOULD NEVER REACH ANYTHING BETTER."*
> —FLORENCE NIGHTINGALE

My applications were in for law school, I had no thoughts of being a nurse. But as my father had famously quoted over the years: "Life is what happens to you when you are busy making other plans" (John Lennon). I should have been better prepared for what happened.

I was out to dinner with my mom, in what I thought was a celebration of my future law school direction when she said, "We don't think you should be an attorney; you should be a nurse."

I found myself staring incredulously across the table, my brain struggling to process the words that came out of her mouth. I had a recollection of her phone call from a few short years before, telling me she had been accepted to nursing school at the age of 49, and asking me, "Am I too old to go?" "Of course not!" I responded. My mom had always dreamed of being a nurse and she became a brilliant one. I, on the other hand, had firm plans to go to law school. "Mom, I love you, but I don't want to do what you do—the long hours of death, disease, and exhaustion—just not for me." And it was then she spoke the words that forever altered my future: "There are many strong attorneys in the world; we need more strong nurses. We need new nurses with different views to save the profession—we need you as a nurse."

At the time, I was working on a presidential campaign and healthcare was a big topic on the campaign trail—although not as central as it became years later. I recognized the truth in her statement, as in all my time on the campaign trail, I had met many attorneys discussing healthcare, but not one nurse that I could recall at all the events. And it seemed to me, how can others make policies regarding healthcare when they had little to no direct knowledge of the situation?

I agreed to apply to one nursing school. I was told at my nursing school interview there was a 2-year waiting list. Feeling relieved that I had held up my end of the bargain and would be heading to law school, I was shocked when 2 weeks later, I received an acceptance letter for nursing school to start in the fall. Realizing fate has a funny way of changing one's plans, I took the acceptance as a sign I was to be a nurse.

Nursing was everything and nothing like I had expected. From nursing school to practice, there has never been anything more challenging I have ever faced professionally—moments of incredible triumph of passing a nursing school exam to saving a life, to incredible feelings of voicelessness and disempowerment as simply being "just a nurse" in the hierarchical design of healthcare. And it was this feeling of disempowerment, lack of ability to drive change, lack of impact on an outcome for a patient and my nursing students, and a strong sense of discontentment that gave me the catalyst I needed to start my first company, HireNurses.com.

"*Were there none who were discontented, the world would never reach anything better*"— Florence Nightingale. Who knew Flo had defined entrepreneurship along with nursing 200 years earlier?

I was working as a hospice nurse practitioner in March 2013 when a patient told me that she was moving to a nursing home because their family couldn't find affordable care to keep her at home. She was devastated. I left my morning visit feeling deflated and headed back to my community college office where I worked as professor of nursing. I was meeting with seven of my former students who had graduated in December 2012 and had yet to find a nursing job; the desperation in the air was palpable. They had consistently been told, "Become a nurse; you will always have a job." I was meeting with them to rewrite their resumes when I turned to the Internet to search for a website that could help them find nursing jobs. Finding none, I reflected on my own experience of searching for a nursing job and the feeling of each sent resume falling into a black hole. The whole day left me feeling frustrated and depressed, as if I were unable to make a difference in the world.

That night, I woke up from a dead sleep. I knew what I had to do. I turned to my husband, shaking him awake to say, "I have to build a website to help nurses find jobs and those who want to hire nurses." He mumbled something like "that's great," turning back over to sleep. Not receiving the enthusiastic response I had been looking for, I got out of bed and called my favorite nurse, my mother. I got her on the phone, explained to her my idea, and she said, "That's great, but it's the middle of the night, could we talk in the morning?" I think they thought I'd sleep off the idea—but no luck—that morning I was more fired up than ever to get going. It was the beginning of HireNurses.com.

My mother gave me her nursing retirement funds to start HireNurses and for a year of my life I worked 18 hours a day, juggling a regular job and raising three little kids, starting my nights with building HireNurses from 9 p.m. to 2 a.m. with a company based in India. It was a grueling year—what I thought was going to be the hardest year—but it was just the tip of the iceberg. When the website was finally ready and we launched, I assumed the rest would just happen. When nothing did, a random moment of luck and a conversation with a fellow young entrepreneur changed my direction. He told me, "Rebecca, you should attend a healthcare hackathon."

At the time, I had no idea what a hackathon was or how it would forever shape my future, and become a transformative step in my entrepreneurial journey. If you don't know what a hackathon is, don't worry—I didn't either. In a quick summary, a hackathon is a 3-day event where people of all different backgrounds come together to present problems in healthcare they want to solve; people form teams and, over the course of the weekend, come up with new solutions to the problems. It was the most brilliant and exciting event I had ever attended as a nurse, and one I'm not sure I was supposed to be at as I realized shortly upon arrival at the event that I was the only nurse in the room. No one asked me to leave, so I stayed, and over the course of that weekend, I learned more about the business of healthcare than I had learned in a year of trying to start a healthcare business. In addition, what shocked me the most is that my opinion as a nurse was highly valued by my team and the mentors who walked into the room probing our solution as to why it would or would not be a success. I had never experienced such validation of my healthcare knowledge in my nursing career as I did at the hackathon.

This hackathon transformed my view of nursing and the impact we could have on the world of healthcare. The experience made me critically aware that nurses have the practical frontline knowledge to create really great healthcare solutions. I started to study the environment of healthcare hackathons around greater Boston. The more I learned that few nurses attended healthcare hackathons, but that many of the winning teams had nurses on them, I knew nurses were key to winning solutions. I became focused on the idea that there had to be a nurse hackathon.

I finally built up the courage to call my nursing alma mater and I connected with Dr. Nancy Hanrahan who, at the time, was the Dean of Nursing at Northeastern University. I told her about my experience at the hackathon and said to her, "You should host a nurse hackathon." And that is the moment an opportunity was presented that changed the rest of my life. Nancy said, "I'm going to host a Summit on Innovation and Entrepreneurship. Why don't you run a nurse hackathon?" In a split second, I went from thinking "I've been to a hackathon" to "Sure, I'll run a hackathon." And from that day forward, for every day for nearly a year of my life, I volunteered my time toward building the event with an incredible team of others who also came forward to donate their time and resources to make the first "Nurse Innovation and Entrepreneurship Summit and Nurse Hackathon" happen in June 2016.

I cannot express enough the importance of volunteering—if I had never volunteered, I would never have advanced along my path of innovation and entrepreneurship. Volunteering provides you the opportunity to shine and deliver in a way no one will offer you in your current career position. Unfortunately, few are going to see your talents when you are doing your normal 12-hour nursing shifts; you are going to have to go the extra mile and volunteer to do more than what is expected of you to show others what you are capable of. Not to mention, volunteering puts you in touch with others who also believe that giving back is central to their mission in life, and those are the kind of people you want to be surrounded by.

I remember a colleague of mine approaching me at my community college and asking, "Why are you spending so much time volunteering on that project? You know they will never hire you." I was shocked—I had never even thought about a new job—I fundamentally wanted there to be a nurse hackathon and to be a part of something bigger, something that would change the future of nursing.

Surprising as it was, volunteering did translate into a new opportunity—I was offered the position as the first Director of Nurse Innovation and Entrepreneurship at Northeastern, which also happened to be the first such role in the United States. In 2 years' time, we ran and participated in 36 events, published 18 publications, and came in contact with the most amazing nurses I have ever met in my career, nurses who have walked on the edge of traditional nursing to create new paths and professions I never knew existed before in nursing.

The program we built was summed up perfectly by Noah Hendler, who said, "We created a place for unicorns," and this tribe of unicorns spoke to my soul.

HireNurses was acquired in March 2018, and I was able to pay my mom back her nursing retirement with some interest, along with several others who had believed in me against the odds, including my right-hand nurse, Faith Lawlor—without either of them I would not have made it. It was one of the proudest days of my life. I had very different plans for where I thought life would go when I started HireNurses, that is, CEO, big office, front page of *Fortune* magazine, and so on, none of which happened. My dad's frequent quoting of John Lennon echoed again: "Life is what happens to you when you are busy making other plans," and once again it had. These unexpected plans led me to the greatest and most rewarding professional experiences of my life. By starting HireNurses, attending a hackathon, and volunteering, my life and future transitioned into being able to help start and lead one of the greatest movements in nursing history: nursing innovation and entrepreneurship.

After transitioning from Northeastern in July 2018, I struggled with a void in my life from the missing tribe of nurses in which I had become associated. In early January 2019, I went for a walk in the bright, frigid, winter air, searching for a New Year's resolution, when the name SONSIEL, The Society of Nurse Scientists, Innovators, Entrepreneurs, and Leaders, came to me. And luckily for me, Dr. Hanrahan and Noah Hendler agreed to give it a go, and together we set out to contact all those incredible nurses we had met before to see whether they would give us their names, titles, and reputations to create a new nursing society—designed to redefine what is possible for nursing. Unbelievably, the first 100 nurses we contacted responded with an overwhelming confirmation of involvement to be founding members of this new organization. At the time of this publication to nearly 8 months later, SONSIEL is an official 501c(3); has hosted the first, sold-out "ThinC: The Healthcare Conference" designed by nurses to advance the best in healthcare; was accepted as an affiliate member of the United Nations to place nurses on committees at the United Nations; has had over 500 inquiries by nurses in 3 months to join SONSIEL; and has hosted our first nurse hackathon supported by Johnson & Johnson on November 15–17, 2019, in New Brunswick, New Jersey. It has been a whirlwind of incredible energy by inspirational nurses who have a vision of a world where nurses are significant leaders recognized for transforming healthcare and our society. Come join us!

Life has a strange way of working out if you decide to bet on yourself. There is so much pressure from society and from nursing to live your career a certain way to achieve "success." Seeing life differently, or taking a different path from the rest, takes a tremendous amount of courage. But this has always been the way for those who have seen the world's potential, rather than its boundaries. Staying true to yourself, your ideals, and your hopes for a better world is a long and often lonely road that may take you to the forefront of failure and thoughts of throwing in the towel, before suddenly the headwinds change and for a moment you realize that although the odds are against you, perhaps you are in fact making progress. There is no one better on earth or with truer intentions to make the world a better place through innovation and entrepreneurship than nurses. Carpe diem!

SUPPLEMENTAL RESOURCES

- HireNurses.com

  https://www.hirenurses.com

- Healthcare Hackathon Database

  http://hackingmedicine.mit.edu/health-hackathon-database

- Northeastern University

  http://catalog.northeastern.edu/undergraduate/health-sciences/nursing

  Director of Nurse Innovation and Entrepreneurship at Northeastern
    - https://www.massdigitalhealth.org/sites/mehi/files/digitalhealth_profile_RebeccaLove_12-12-17.pdf

- Nurse Innovation and Entrepreneurship Summit and Nurse Hackathon

  https://news.northeastern.edu/tag/nurse-innovation-and-entrepreneurship-summit-and-hackathon/

- Nurse Hackathon supported by Johnson & Johnson, November 2019

  https://nursing.jnj.com/nursing-news-events/nurses-hacking-healthcare

- SONSIEL: Society of Nurse Scientists, Innovators, Entrepreneurs, and Leaders

  https://www.sonsiel.com

Shift Disruptors: Stories of Nurses Recognizing Their Unique Role in Healthcare

It's not easy being different—to be a trailblazer, innovator, influencer, or leader. However, just because it isn't easy, doesn't mean it's not possible. We all have a unique story, vision, and understanding about healthcare, health delivery, and patient best practices. Yet, the beauty of the collective voice of nurses is that we are all working toward one goal: to disrupt the status quo and improve life for those around us and those we care for. This chapter displays the stories of such nurses, the early parts of their career, the literal shift that occurred, and the unique voice they each hold. Their stories are still evolving, just like yours. They are the unicorns, the passionate caregivers, the rogue thinkers; they are the shift disruptors and they are nurses.

Nurses Lighting Paths to Healthcare Transformation

STEPHAN DAVIS, DNP, MHSA, NEA-BC, CENP, CNE, FACHE, FIEL

> "*DARKNESS CANNOT DRIVE OUT DARKNESS, ONLY LIGHT CAN DO THAT.*"
> —DR. MARTIN LUTHER KING, JR.

A bright ray of light illuminated the unexplored corners of my mind. That is the best way I can describe the moment I was inspired to become a nurse. I was 18 years old, studying music in New York City, realizing an aspiration for which I prepared a decade. Living in New York for only a few months, however, transformed my thinking and further developed a passion for equality and social justice. After realizing that music alone would not provide the platform I wanted to create change in the world, a quote from Martin Luther King, Jr., ultimately led me to the path I am on today. Dr. King argued that "of all the forms of inequality, injustice in healthcare is the most shocking and inhuman." Reflecting on King's words, I was moved to contribute to the healthcare system's transformation—to actualize a reimagined infrastructure that provides for, protects, and includes all people.

This desire to improve health for all people has guided my professional and academic pursuits in nursing and healthcare leadership. My time in graduate school at Georgetown University reaffirmed my inspiration. In the spirit of Jesuit tradition, Georgetown teaches its graduates to be "women and men for others." This mission led me to join a project providing didactic and experiential learning opportunities to unemployed District of Columbia residents, in order to prepare them for employment opportunities at local hospitals. It moved me to become a volunteer nurse at Whitman-Walker in Washington, DC, and to later serve on the board at APICHA Community Health Center in New York City—both organizations that provide care to minorities and socioeconomically disadvantaged populations. It has inspired me to lead healthcare organizations to achieve designations in healthcare equality, which symbolize a commitment to diversity and inclusion for patients and healthcare professionals. Finally, it guided my decision to pursue doctoral education at Yale University, School of Nursing, the nation's first collegiate school of nursing, whose founding mission is "better health for all people."

In my career, I have cared for patients, led diverse organizations, and served on various boards and task forces. During my time at Yale, I underwent a professional transformation. I served as the executive director of professional practice, overseeing organizational learning, nursing quality, and clinical excellence initiatives. Developing people, bridging partnerships between academia and practice, and advancing diversity and inclusion gave me the greatest satisfaction in this position. By this point, I was no longer satisfied with working for only one organization; rather, I wanted to help advance these issues at state and national levels. Academia would likely provide me with the rich milieu within which I could explore my greatest passions.

After a decade of advancing healthcare leadership within acute care organizations, I made the transition to academia. I now serve as clinical assistant professor and liaison for clinical agencies and innovative partnerships at Georgia State University, where I teach courses in nursing leadership, management, and policy. From 2017 through 2019, I also served as an elected board director for the Georgia Nurses Association's leadership development initiatives, fostering the leadership capacity of more than 100,000 nurses in the state. At a national level, I have given talks and seminars at prestigious organizations, including Vanderbilt University Medical Center, Children's Hospital of Philadelphia, Northwestern Medicine, and the American College of Healthcare Executives (ACHE). Through my teaching and service as a fellow and national faculty member of ACHE—the leading professional society for healthcare management—I have guided and professionally developed members and fellows across the nation. I have also had the privilege of serving as a leadership committee member of ACHE's LGBT Forum, a group dedicated to advancing diversity and inclusion for the LGBT patient population and members of the healthcare workforce. Building upon my prior work involving the intersection of education, diversity and inclusion, and professional development for leaders, I am currently pursuing a doctor of education degree in mind, brain, and teaching at Johns Hopkins University. My doctoral research will focus on explicit and implicit bias affecting gender and sexual minorities among current and aspiring healthcare professionals. In my relatively short career, I have had the opportunity to pursue many different interests that center upon my core mission to advance health for all people. I have worked with extraordinary people, led projects that have expanded hearts and minds, and contributed to the professional development of leaders across the nation.

As a healthcare leader and educator, I am continuously inspired by the unique strengths and contributions of those who provide care and who seek care within our healthcare community—the environmental services professional who has worked at the hospital for 30 years, whom patients mention by name; the physical therapist who pushes patients to walk when they feel they are not ready, helping people to achieve more than they believed was possible; the oncology patients, who despite their prognosis, wake up to fight each and every day; and, whether serving in clinical, education, research, or leadership roles, I am inspired by the millions of nurses whose collective work represents the most trusted profession in America.

Throughout my journey in healthcare, I have encountered extraordinary nurses who are advancing professional practice and clinical care delivery every day. My first chief nursing officer, Dr. Lisa Rowen, led the University of Maryland Medical Center to improve health outcomes and achieve Magnet designation. A team of nurse-scientists I worked with as a graduate assistant at Georgetown developed a capacity-building intervention to increase the skills of nurses in Africa who provide autonomous care within countries most devastated by the HIV/AIDS epidemic. Jill Case-Wirth, the chief nurse executive for WellStar Health System, led the organization to create innovative care models that include clinical nurse leaders and clinical nurse specialists at a time when many health systems either do not utilize or underutilize these important roles. Laurie Fugitt successfully advocated for a change in Georgia law that allowed naloxone to be administered without a prescription in order to prevent overdose. These nurses have inspired me with their unrelenting efforts to advance health and professional nursing practice.

In addition, there are nurses who contribute to healthcare transformation through entrepreneurship and innovation, as well as regional and national leadership. Joe Novello is the founder of NurseGrid, a mobile application that is changing how nurses in direct care roles communicate with each other and their unit leaders. Dr. Michelle Nelson, president of two APRN associations, had the vision to unify nurses in all areas of practice. In 2018, she led the development of the inaugural Unity Conference for Nursing Excellence, which featured clinicians, legislators, educators, scholars, and executives across the state of Georgia, as well as national leaders such as Dr. Ernest Grant, the first man to become president of the American Nurses Association (ANA). Lastly,

Dr. Ken White, renowned educator, executive, and author, led the charge within the ACHE to create an ACHE member group for LGBT healthcare executives and allies to advance diversity and inclusion for the LGBT patient population and workforce. In 2019, Dr. White became the first openly gay man to receive ACHE's Gold Medal Award, the highest honor in the field of healthcare management.

I could go on and on about the exceptional nurse leaders, educators, researchers, and clinicians who have helped me keep my fire burning brightly for our profession. The fight of millions of other nurses, just as extraordinary as my friends and colleagues, who are working diligently to advance health for patients and populations here and abroad, nourishes me with the hope I need to continue working to transform the healthcare system. Just as Florence Nightingale, affectionately referred to as "the lady with the lamp," lit the way forward for our profession, I believe that all nurses have the capacity to light new paths, which will ultimately lead us to reform the healthcare system and actualize reimagined care delivery. Yet, for some of us, complex challenges, fear, and insecurity dampen our spark that could ignite change in the world around us. At times, seemingly insurmountable obstacles overwhelm and discourage us, and we lose sight of all that is at stake—which is, ultimately, the fulfillment of our personal and collective missions. I, too, know this struggle. When I experience these times, I often reflect on a quote from the book *A Return to Love*, which moves me when darkness looms over my light:

> *Our deepest fear is not that we are inadequate. Our deepest fear is that we are powerful beyond measure. It is our light not our darkness that most frightens us. We ask ourselves, who am I to be brilliant, gorgeous, talented and fabulous? Actually, who are you not to be? …Your playing small does not serve this world. …We are all meant to shine, as children do. … And as we let our own light shine, we unconsciously give others permission to do the same (Williamson, 1992, p. 190).*

So it has become my mission to encourage and help all nurses and all healthcare professionals and leaders to use their unique gifts, talents, and strengths in order to shine brilliantly in places in which darkness shrouds. Each and every patient expects this of us. The healthcare system relies upon us for this reason. With our light, we each hold the power to inspire and make change, even in the face of adversity. And together, we will light the paths to healthcare transformation—for our communities, the nation, and the world.

SUPPLEMENTAL RESOURCES

- Georgetown University, School of Nursing and Health Studies
  https://nhs.georgetown.edu/degree-programs
- Volunteer with WWH: Whitman-Walker Health
  https://www.whitman-walker.org/volunteer
- APICHA Community Health Center in New York City
  https://www.apicha.org
- Yale University, School of Nursing
  https://nursing.yale.edu
- Georgia State University, School of Nursing
  https://nursing.gsu.edu
- Georgia Nurses Association
  https://georgianurses.nursingnetwork.com/?endorse=gna

- ACHE: The American College of Healthcare Executives
  https://www.ache.org
- ACHE LGBT Forum
  https://www.ache.org/membership/forums-and-networks/lgbt-forum
- Johns Hopkins University, School of Nursing
  https://nursing.jhu.edu
- WellStar Health System
  https://www.wellstar.org/pages/default.aspx
- Governor Deal signs naloxone bill into law—expanding access to an emergency tool to parents to help fight opioid epidemic
  https://gdna.georgia.gov/press-releases/2017-06-26/governor-deal-signs-naloxone-bill-law-expanding-access-emergency-tool
- NurseGrid
  https://nursegrid.com
- United Advanced Practice Registered Nurses of Georgia, 2019 Annual Unity Conference for Nursing Excellence
  https://uaprn.enpnetwork.com/nurse-practitioner-events/126161-2019-annual-unity-conference#!info
- American Nurses Association (ANA)
  https://www.nursingworld.org

Overcoming Obstacles to Find My Voice

AMY ROSE TAYLOR, AGNP-BC, BSN, RN

"THE ART OF NURSING IS MORE THAN A GENTLE TOUCH OR A WELL-TIMED SMILE.... IT'S THE ABILITY TO ADVOCATE FOR OUR PATIENTS AS WELL AS ADVOCATING FOR OUR PEERS."

My quiet life and career in human resources was disrupted when my mother was diagnosed with breast cancer. I became her support, accompanying her to countless doctor's appointments, screenings, evaluations, and surgeries. Through five lumpectomies, a double mastectomy, and several reconstructive surgeries, I learned how to change her bandages, attend to her drains, and provide her with the emotional support needed to cope with the loss of the most outward sign of her femininity.

The months I spent with her in and out of the hospital inspired me to take a different path from the one I was on. I set out to become a nurse, taking the prerequisite classes in order to enroll in nursing school. But before my schooling was complete, I experienced nursing from the patient's perspective. In early 2011, I delivered my fourth child. During the course of my pregnancy, a doctor discovered a lump in my right breast. He assured me that it was probably nothing, but encouraged me to follow up with a breast surgeon. Where I had once been the comforting presence attending to my mother as she fought breast cancer, the positions quickly reversed as one test after another indicated my need to undergo a double mastectomy.

Even though I was advised to delay my classes until after I had time to heal, I found that the courses I was taking became an outlet during this challenging period of time. When I could no longer stand to read one more article about living with breast cancer or the possibilities offered by alternative treatments, I could read my textbooks with relish. Aiding my mother gave me the desire to be a nurse and the confidence to know that I could help someone after a devastating loss. It wasn't until I had experienced these major life changes that I discovered how much I adored the art of nursing.

Nursing is both an art and a science. We study the science of it, spend hours learning the pathophysiology of disease and healing and the intricacies of pharmacokinetics, and can write care plans until our fingers are numb. We understand the "HOW" of the disease process so that we can answer when our patients ask us, "HOW COME THIS HAPPENED TO ME?" That's where the art of nursing comes in. We have to skillfully and deftly answer our patients who are struggling with a diagnosis, tactfully answer a family's questions about a prognosis, and tenderly offer advice to patients who might not be willing to listen. The art of nursing is more than a gentle touch or a well-timed smile; it's the ability to juggle multiple patients' needs simultaneously during a 12-hour shift, when you may not have time to sit down. It's the ability to work within a team environment and bring a nursing perspective to a roundtable discussion. It's the ability to advocate for our patients as well as advocating for our peers.

When I entered my nursing program, I was a single mom who was struggling to raise four children under the age of 10. Today, I am married with five children, and I enjoy my position as a geriatric nurse practitioner for UnitedHealth Group. Many people have asked me how I managed to juggle the responsibilities of a family with the rigorous requirements of a full-time nursing program, and my response has been that failure was not an option. When I thought I couldn't study for one more minute, or write one more paper, I would look at my children and know that I had to go on. My family was depending on me to succeed and I wouldn't let them down.

During my master's degree studies, I was accepted as the Health Policy Fellow for the American Association of Nurse Practitioners. As the Fellow, I worked in Washington, DC, on Capitol Hill, and I was able to see firsthand how much we have accomplished as nurses—and how much further we have to go. I urge all nurses to remain advocates for our profession, both at home and with our elected officials. You don't have to attend a Lobby Day, write letters to your elected officials, or remain active in your respective professional organizations, but that certainly does help. As advocates, we must remember that we represent the more than 3 million nurses nationwide, and 250,000 nurse practitioners. Everything we do reflects on the public's perception of our skill and ability, so we wear our white coats with pride as leaders in our field. Working as a Fellow helped clarify the challenges that we face as nurses, as well as the need to present a united voice on behalf of our patients. There is a reason why nursing is considered to be the most trusted profession, and we must leverage that trust to speak for those who cannot speak for themselves.

Following my experience as a Fellow, I decided that the best way to utilize my skills was to write a book about becoming a nurse, in order to encourage the next generation of nurses to follow suit. And that's what I did. I spent my time writing *Nursing School 101* in the evenings and on weekends, trying to put my knowledge into print to inspire others to follow into this field. In writing the book, I learned that, as a nurse, we don't always have to be at the bedside to inspire others or to drive change. Nurses are an integral part of our healthcare system, and as such, we aren't always the ones dressed in scrubs or giving out medications. Sometimes, we are the ones who are at the forefront of change, driving innovation, breaking down barriers, and building bridges with our many colleagues in healthcare.

At this time, I work as a geriatric provider for Optum, a division of UnitedHealth Group. I see members in their homes and work as a part of an interdisciplinary team to bring care to the most disadvantaged persons. I advocate for my patients, not only within our healthcare system for preapprovals and out of network providers, but also outside in the community with our nonprofit partners, trying to get their basic needs met. I am also the voice of the company's podcast, Clinician Commons Live, where I interview fellow employees and inspiring people in healthcare. Each week, tens of thousands of people tune in to listen to my stories and hear my interviews. I use my voice as a platform to get people to start thinking about change and innovation and to strategize ways to improve health for all.

It is a very exciting time to be a nurse or a nurse practitioner. We are watching the medical system transform every day, from a system in which solo practitioners would make house calls and handwrite their prescriptions, to one in which healthcare is a team effort and technology is increasingly integrated into care. As nurses, we are in the middle of that change, providing care, conducting research, and integrating evidence-based practice for the betterment of our patients. As nurses, we have been given the skills and the training necessary to lead the way. I never expected my mother's cancer to springboard me into this position, but this experience has allowed me to utilize my skills as an advocate, a provider, and a storyteller to benefit my patients and my profession.

SUPPLEMENTAL RESOURCES

- UnitedHealth Group
  https://www.unitedhealthgroup.com
- Optum, UnitedHealth Group
  https://www.unitedhealthgroup.com/businesses/optum.html
- Fellows Program at the American Association of Nurse Practitioners
  https://www.aanp.org/membership/fellows-program

Kaizen at Massachusetts General Hospital

HIYAM M. NADEL, RN, MBA, CGC

"I BEGAN TO REALIZE THAT THIS WAS AN OPPORTUNITY TO SHOWCASE WHAT NURSING CAN CONTRIBUTE, BECAUSE NURSES ACTUALLY ARE IN THE BEST POSITION TO UNDERSTAND PATIENT AND STAFF WORKFLOW."

You know you are different. You see and think in such different ways, most of the time no one else can see the way you perceive things. My father told me that I used to scare him when, at 9 years of age, I would wake up in the mornings and say things like "Dad, I know what causes cancer; it's the excessive use of pesticides on everything we eat." Although that theory didn't explain everything, years later evidence would come out that certain chemicals and pesticides are in fact carcinogenic. This example, among others, made my father believe I would surely end up as a PhD researcher or a physician.

Being a first-generation college student in an immigrant family from a war-torn country was difficult. It took all I had to work nights after attending classes all day. The thought of going to graduate or medical school seemed too daunting. How could I possibly make the money to achieve that? My family was poor and bank loans seemed impossible. I won several monetary awards in high school but used that money to pay off my family's bills, so I could focus on my coursework. Luckily, I did get loans through undergraduate school, established credit, then financed my education, but everything was a struggle.

Although medical school was my goal, I signed up for nursing instead, thinking I could work as a nurse to earn money, make up classes in the summer to complete the biology major, then eventually go to medical school. But, the high touch point with patients and their families made me fall in love with nursing. Throughout the nursing program, while doing co-op work in various hospitals, I would devise or create work-arounds for patient care. Much later, I would see my ideas implemented as a real product on the market. I wondered: what prevented me from completing the loop from idea to marketable product on my own? This internal questioning continued to bother me and motivate me to find an answer. However, the need to support myself and family obligations got in the way.

As my experience in nursing began to grow, ideas came at a faster pace, yet I was unable to act on them due to the rigorous nature of my day-to-day job. Switching from inpatient to outpatient was a defining moment, as it provided me the leeway to take the next step.

My specialty is women's health, specifically OB/GYN with an expertise in maternal-fetal medicine. Because of this expertise, I was recruited, along with five physicians, to reopen the obstetrics department at Massachusetts General Hospital (MGH) after a 42-year hiatus. I initially agreed to start on a consultative basis only, as I was afraid that the entire project would fail.

The moment I walked through the doors of MGH, it became clear it was a very special place. The excitement was palpable among the executive obstetrics committee, with discussions around the table that were passionate but respectful. The committee included nurses, as well as physicians and administrators. Prior to this, I experienced little, if any, nursing involvement or contribution at this level. My assessment was confirmed when the chief nursing officer introduced me to the architects so that there would be direct nursing input regarding the design of the ambulatory practice, labor and delivery, the operating rooms, and the postpartum floors.

This was a much greater responsibility than I had previously borne, and I felt I had so much more to prove as a nurse. But I began to realize that this was an opportunity to showcase what nursing can contribute, because nurses actually are in the best position to understand patient and staff workflow. I was convinced that this was the time to think outside the box. I began to observe patient and staff movement; implemented time studies to understand time wasted in the system; and devised a nursing care model.

Several months into the planning phase, I also knew this was where I wanted to be employed. Having visionary leaders as my mentors, my creative side resurfaced, and I now had the confidence to discuss this novel nurse model when I was offered the opportunity to stay as the leader of the ambulatory division. Facing a lukewarm response, I was given 2 years to prove my model, with a parting of ways with no hard feelings if it didn't work. My vision was successful, and I remained employed in the department for over 2 decades.

In the ambulatory division, I quickly came to realize that one must see medical practice as a business, and obstetrics became our "start-up." I made sure I was involved in every aspect of the practice: clinical, marketing, human resources, operations, finance, and billing. All of these were critical dimensions to understanding and running "the business."

Subsequently, I became intimately involved in expanding our practice with different subspecialties at multiple sites. I was also involved in creating our own electronic medical record and other information technology products, a forerunner of today's ubiquitous instruments. I have done things I would never have had an opportunity to do, had I not taken a leap of faith to work at MGH. Furthermore, I had the opportunity to be involved in every aspect of running a practice, rather than allowing myself to get pigeonholed into certain tasks.

Having been lucky enough to prove my mettle in such an innovative and collaborative institution, I was invited to work on many varied projects, which in turn led to my getting recruited to work in those same fields. Since I did so many build outs, I was recruited by an architectural firm; and because of my finance and billing knowledge, I was recruited by one of the top six accounting firms. I stayed at MGH, but this led me to conclude that I could contribute in many meaningful ways.

With the entrepreneurial juices flowing, when our family friend asked if we would get involved in his idea of an incontinence device, I jumped at the idea. We currently have a company, and at the time of this writing, clinical trials at several sites are on-going (fingers crossed).

In 2016, MGH began giving two annual Innovation Design Excellence Awards of $5,000 each. These grants are designed to encourage nurses and other health professionals to think creatively about problems they encounter on a daily basis, and consider how their solutions could be implemented in a larger context. We have been pleasantly surprised at the number of applications and wonderful ideas. I have been lucky to serve as the awardees' mentor in developing their ideas; several prototypes have been realized, addressing problems such as patient falls, pressure ulcers, and central line infection prevention.

Now I am about to embark on a new chapter in my career, which I believe to be the most important, since it will have a wider impact. In September, I will become Director for the Center of Innovation in patient care delivery at MGH. In this new role, I hope to build an infrastructure for both nurses and other direct caregivers to promote idea generation and implementation of creative solutions to clinical problems. Our goal is to make patient care more effective, easier to implement, safer, less unpleasant for the patient, and less expensive. This has certain parallels to the Japanese concept of *kaizen*, or continuous improvement, which has been so successfully implemented by Toyota Motor Corporation, where everyone in the company is encouraged to creatively solve problems.

The nurses I have worked with so far have told me they want to stay at the bedside in caring for patients, because they now have a creative outlet when they see their ideas coming to fruition. They gain, the patients gain, and the organization gains. And I have come full circle: from frustration at being unable to implement my ideas, to the satisfaction of enabling others to create and implement theirs.

SUPPLEMENTAL RESOURCES

- Massachusetts General Hospital
  https://www.massgeneral.org
- Innovation Design Excellence Awards
  https://www.massgeneral.org/research/news/Nursing-Research/nursing-IDEA.aspx
- The Magic of Kaizen
  https://www.americannursetoday.com/magic-kaizen
- Carroll, W. M. (2020). *Emerging technologies for nurses: Implications for practice*. New York, NY: Springer Publishing Company.

Nurse Superheroes

MARION LEARY, MSN, MPH, RN

"ALTHOUGH IT TOOK A WHILE TO FIND MY ORIGIN STORY, AND MY WAY TO NURSING, LIFE IS NEVER ONE EASY-TO-FOLLOW PATH, AS IS THE CASE WITH RESEARCH AND INNOVATION."

I have what I like to call a superhero complex. I believe that I have certain superpowers that most other people do not: like the Flash I am fast—I walk fast, I work fast, I drive fast; like Daredevil—I see problems differently than most people, ultimately solving them through spirited innovation; and like Superman—I can bring people back from the dead, though not by circling the Earth so fast that it spins in an opposite rotation.

This obsession with being a superhero began when I was young. My twin sister and I were very much into reading comic books, watching superhero cartoons, and playing with superhero action figures. One night, we dressed up in homemade superhero costumes to go out into the night to fight crime. After much debate, however, we realized we would get into a lot of trouble if our parents found out we climbed out of our second floor bedroom window into the darkness below. It was a very short-lived double life! Even now, I still love a superhero flick—the Avengers, Supergirl, all the Marvel movies, and some DC movies.

Looking back, what drew me to superheroes was the altruism of saving lives and the science and technology used to enhance their super powers. When I was young, being a geek was not a trait that was particularly celebrated by my peers. It wasn't until my late 20s that I began to embrace my geekiness. With these social challenges, I struggled to figure out what I wanted to be when I grew up. I could have never imagined the superpowers I would obtain by becoming an academic resuscitation scientist and nurse innovator.

It was during my high school years when my fascination with saving lives became the calling I knew I had to pursue. I became an emergency medical technician and loved getting up in the middle of the night, putting on my uniform, and racing out to help others in distress. It was almost the same thing as dressing up in a superhero costume and going to fight crime—except I didn't have to climb out of my bedroom window and I wasn't going to get in trouble for doing it! After High School, I started working for a number of nonprofit organizations, trying to find my path and passion. Once I finally went to college, I switched majors more than a few times. It wasn't until I saw an advertisement for a nurse research program at a local university that I remembered my passion for science and saving lives.

Although my family members were not college-educated, I went on to receive two master's degrees from an Ivy League institution and I am currently in a doctoral program. For all intents and purposes, I am as alien to my family as Kal-El (aka Superman) was to the Kents or Kara Zor-El (aka Supergirl) was to the Danvers.

With their love and support though, I became a critical care nurse—resuscitating more people than I care to remember—and then a resuscitation scientist, where I perform the research and write the science behind the CPR guidelines. Through the creation of these innovative solutions for sudden cardiac arrest, I have found a new set of skills and passions to

(Adapted from a Medium post: For the love of (superheroes) and science, performed at the Philadelphia Science Festival storytelling event.)

bring to my new role as the Director of Innovation at the University of Pennsylvania's School of Nursing. I think of each community of nurse innovators as the Avengers—creating new technologies and solutions to the world's toughest problems!

Biomedical research and the many Science, Technology, Engineering, Mathematics (STEM) and Science Technology, Engineering, Art, and Mathematics (STEAM) fields continue to fuel my lifelong fascination for all things science. Over the past decade, I have dedicated my life to spreading their influence to the masses by writing articles and blogs, hosting podcasts, amplifying my voice—and others' voices—on social media, and speaking with students around the country. A couple of years ago, when science was under attack, I came together with a Justice League of dedicated scientists, science communicators, educators, and friends of science from around the globe, to take a stand against evil through the conception and production of the March for Science. As Uncle Ben Parker said to Peter Parker (aka Spiderman): "With great power comes great responsibility." As "science superheroes," we have a responsibility to make a difference and, like Professor X, to teach the next generation of *Gifted Youngsters*.

Although it took a while to find my origin story, and my way to nursing, life is never one easy-to-follow path, as is the case with research and innovation. Today, I work with a group of passionate interdisciplinary colleagues using innovative technology in a lair of my own to save lives—finally embracing the superhero I've been all along.

SUPPLEMENTAL RESOURCES

- Nurses Are Superheroes (Ms. Career Girl)
  http://www.mscareergirl.com/nurses-are-superheroes
- Superhero Nurse Brightens Children's Hospital Stay
  https://nursing.jnj.com/nursing-news-events/superhero-nurse-brightens-childrens-hospital-stay
- Center for Resuscitation Science
  https://resuscitationscience.com
  https://www.med.upenn.edu/resuscitation
- The American Heart Association CPR & ECC
  https://cpr.heart.org/AHAECC/CPRAndECC/UCM_473161_CPR-and-ECC.jsp?_requestid=29807
- The March for Science
  https://marchforscience.com
- Philadelphia Science Festival
  https://www.fi.edu/psf
- For the Love of (Superheroes) and Science
  https://medium.com/@marionleary/for-the-love-of-superheros-and-science-236e1bb5a769

Phoenix Rising

VERONICA SOUTHERLAND, MSN, APRN, FNP-BC

"DOUBT KILLS MORE DREAMS THAN FAILURE EVER WILL. ..."

I was standing at the nurses' station in tears, responsible for a 40-year-old female patient recovering from a quadruple vessel coronary artery bypass graft who was circling the drain fast, and I couldn't get in contact with the surgeon to ask what he wanted me to do next. Then it hit me—if you don't do something, this lady is going to die! The ultimate feeling that things are not in our control can be quite overwhelming, something I knew all too well. As a new nurse at this point in my career, I didn't know it all, but I knew enough to keep going, because this patient needs me. I called all hands on deck in the unit—the charge nurse, house supervisor, another surgeon, multiple others—to help me get through this without my patient dying.

After many years in the emergency department, with days and nights filled with this feeling, I searched for a way to make a change. I realized that the "frequent flyers" of the ED were there because they were not receiving proper care at home. I decided to open a homecare agency, where I could make an impact on patient's lives before their needs evolved into intensive care. We opened in 2006 and within a year and a half we had made our first million, then $2 million by year 2. The money started rolling in. My husband at the time took responsibility for the financials, and I handled the clinical portion with our team of over 200 employees who serviced our six offices across two states. We continued to grow and build relationships. Our reputation in the community was stellar. I learned very quickly to focus on what you can do well, and not on what you can't. Rather than advertising, we relied on referrals from physicians and other healthcare professionals with whom I had previously worked. Before I knew it, we were at $4 million in revenue.

Then, our economy took a nosedive. The new Obamacare initiative was released, the real estate market crashed, and small businesses now had to provide major medical insurance for all of their full-time employees, rather than partial, as we had done in the past. The monthly medical cost for a company of our size was in the six-figure range and our clientele were suffering financially, so they could no longer afford our services. Things got hard, quickly, and I found myself using my personal savings to make payroll every week. I had to lay off over 200 employees and close offices. I was responsible for the livelihood of all these families and I convinced myself that I single-handedly ruined their lives. The emotional strain on myself, not to mention my 20-year marriage, was almost unbearable. We had just built a $1.7 million dollar home that I could no longer afford, my daughter was in private school, and my husband, who had left corporate America to come work in our business, was also now unemployed. Finding work during this time was difficult for him because jobs were few and far between in every industry, regardless of a person's educational background.

I had to do something. So, I worked three jobs and went back to school to pursue my advanced nursing degree, and all the while my 20-year marriage fell apart under the pressure from trying to hold it all together—trying to be a wife, a mother, and a student. I dusted myself off and tried again, because failure was not an option. I could not give up, quit, or be stagnant. I had already lost everything, so what else could possibly happen besides rising from the ashes? As I worked as a nurse practitioner to gain experience after finishing grad school, I knew that I could rise again. I returned and looked at where I could rebuild. I opened my own practice and started doing intravenous hydration. To my amazement, things took off rapidly, and before long, I was being requested to help others get started in the industry.

Today, I own and operate a primary care/urgent care direct patient care model practice, a pain management practice, a hydration lounge, and classes teaching intravenous hydration business startup across the country. It has been a whirlwind of a journey, one during which I have learned a lot about myself, as a nursing innovator and an entrepreneur. Never stop!

SUPPLEMENTAL RESOURCES

- Hansen-Turton, T., Sherman, S., King, E. S. (2015). *Nurse-Led Health Clinics: Operations, Policy, and Opportunities.* New York, NY: Springer Publishing Company.
- Visser, L. S., Montejano, A. S. (2019). *Fast Facts for the Triage Nurse: An Orientation and Care Guide* (2nd ed.).
- Campo, T. M. (2016). *Essential Procedures for Emergency, Urgent, and Primary Care Settings: A Clinical Companion* (2nd ed.). New York, NY: Springer Publishing Company.

"Just a Nurse" With CEO Added to Her Name

BRITTANY MOLKENTHIN, BSN, RN, CPN

"As nurses, we sit at the forefront of changing patients' lives. Our intuitions and passions lead us on the pathway of innovating and improving the lives of others."

Midwife, lactation consultant, maybe an OB/GYN? Labor and delivery nurse, women's health nurse practitioner? Flash forward—pediatric intensive care registered nurse, pediatric primary care nurse practitioner master's candidate, nurse entrepreneur, and CEO. *Wait, how did I get here?* They say in nursing school you'll have patients whom you'll never forget. Many key moments and patients become pivotal in your nursing career. These people and interactions form the foundations of your future.

I chose to shadow a lactation consultant my junior year of nursing school, as an atypical experience that still coincided with my strong passion for maternal–fetal health. Through multiple consults with new breastfeeding mothers on a labor and delivery unit, one mother, just one, resonates in my mind. I walked into the delivery room to find a new mom in her early 20s holding her newborn baby. She was elated, holding her son and staring at him in awe. It's difficult to put the feelings, emotions, and love in the room into words. She excitedly shared her goal to breastfeed her baby, mentioning the many classes she took, how important it was to her, and how eager she was to try.

She placed her baby at her breast with the help of the lactation consultant and shifted positions several times. Nothing seemed to be comfortable, but the lactation consultant assured her this was a normal feeling in the beginning. The baby started to squirm, becoming fussy, as the mom couldn't seem to get the right latch. Tears began to swell in the mother's eyes as she needed to understand what she was doing wrong, "Is he drinking anything?" I felt helpless in the corner. I had no idea if she was doing it right. After all, how can you tell? The baby appeared to breastfeed for what seemed like 30 seconds. The lactation consultant said to give it some time and we would return to help her try again. An hour later, we were back. It progressively worsened—the baby screaming, the mom in hysterics, and I, still helpless, sitting in the corner. To make matters worse, the doctor glanced in and asked how the baby was doing breastfeeding. The mom screamed for formula; she just wanted her baby to eat, she said. She didn't want to be a bad mom and starve him. Refusing to breastfeed again, she cried and bottle-fed her baby, while telling her partner that she was already failing as her baby's mom.

That night, I continuously reflected on this experience. *Was there anything I could have done to help this mom? Why isn't there a method of showing breastfeeding mothers how much breast milk their baby is receiving?* If only I could have helped her, told her how much her baby was receiving. Her birth and breastfeeding experience could have been completely different. After this night, I tucked away this memory and its wrenching feelings, into the back recesses of my mind.

When I was a student at the University of Connecticut (UCONN), the Healthcare Innovations Program was mandatory. We were asked to think of one way that we could improve the healthcare field. If we could make any device to improve the well-being of our patients, what would it be? Many nursing students felt this was an unfair question as we were not even bedside nurses yet. How could nursing students create a business plan with no business background?

As I reflected on my bedside experiences, a light bulb went off in my head. My encounter with the breastfeeding mother suddenly came to the forefront. What if I developed a device that accurately calculated the amount of breast milk that infants receive during breastfeeding? A device that helps the 50% of moms who stop breastfeeding within 2 weeks postpartum because of the apprehension and anxiety that their infant is not receiving enough breast milk, the 60% of moms who do not meet their personal breastfeeding goals, and the drop-off of women who successfully breastfeed their infants—only 25% out of the 84% of women who initiate breastfeeding at birth exclusively breastfeed through 6 months (Office of the Surgeon General, 2011).

I worked with a team of biomedical engineers to develop this device—a working prototype that calculates breast milk intake of the breastfeeding infant in a safe, noninvasive, convenient way. The sensor, using medical grade technology, calculates the amount of breast milk an infant consumes while breastfeeding. Infants will wear the Manoula onesie or strap, mothers will place the Manoula sensor in the pocket that lies over the stomach, and as the baby begins to breastfeed, the sensor calculates direct intake. As a part of the program, it was now time for our Shark Tank-style event at UCONN, where I would pitch the idea and the prototype in hopes of winning the competition. I really wanted to get an A on the paper, but more importantly, I wanted to win the competition. I vividly remember my excitement as I envisioned my victory; I was the only one with a working prototype. Joke was on me, because I lost; I didn't even place. But a good grade was enough at that point.

I went home and reflected on my experience, unable to shake my disappointment. Even more so, one of the judges I encountered from my experience, Kevin Bouley, a distinguished alumnus in UCONN business and engineering, asked questions that made me doubt the value of my device: about a patent search, market penetration, and the product's project revenue costs and regulatory pathway. These queries were a foreign language to me. Nevertheless, I researched Kevin's email, reached out to him, and ultimately changed the entire outlook of my future career in nursing.

I met with Kevin the following day and we discussed my plans for the device. *Was this something I could actually bring to the market? Can I help breastfeeding mothers?* His advice sticks with me to this day, "You know, Brittany, nurses can be innovators, too. And entrepreneurs."

I spent the year after graduation starting the company—an LLC, Lactation Innovations. I worked with a team of lawyers and filed a provisional patent. I learned what it meant to network, what a pitch deck was, and the importance of using LinkedIn. Networking is about forming relationships with others. An advisor of mine once said, "You never know what can come from a conversation." The power of networking—attending events that are in the space of innovation and nursing—helped me build my team, find advisors, and grow the company. The pitch deck is the most important document for a small startup: it is an ever-changing presentation of slides that presents your business plan. It evolves as the company evolves and is used to present to investors, to potential partners, and in competitions. Everyone always asks, "Can you send me over your pitch deck to review?" LinkedIn, a networking site for professionals, can link you to important key players in your field, and help you start those conversations with people who may be doing similar work that you are doing, or with whom you could be potential partners in the future. Some of my best connections came from a simple LinkedIn connection request. I submitted several grants, one being an SBIR (Small Business Innovation Research) grant to the National Institutes of Health (NIH), which was an experience in itself. I kept the company alive, while simultaneously learning what it meant to have a company and be a CEO. This company grew alongside my first bedside job as a pediatric intensive care registered nurse at Connecticut Children's Medical Center and my ongoing studies to become a pediatric primary care nurse practitioner.

Throughout this bustling lifestyle, I quickly learned that I was lacking the right team. In 2018, just over a year later, I hired a chief operating officer, Jayme, who is now my mentor, friend, and business partner. Jayme's background in developing medical devices brings advantageous contributions throughout our many business encounters. Together we have submitted several grants, and bootstrapped and raised monies through grants to further develop the device. Bootstrapping is when founders personally fund their business, and it is very common in the initial stages of the company. Grants are nondilutive funds that help you fund your startup. The government has many grants available to people starting a business. We have launched our website, which promotes exposure on the Internet. It allows you to gain a follower base and helps people get excited about your product and company. We have refined our prototype and began testing for optimization, by analyzing the safety of our device and its capabilities. Prototypes go through a series of stages during development, from a proof of concept, then minimal viable product (MVP) prototype, into an alpha prototype, and so forth. This leads to a product that is production and manufacturing ready. In addition, we established key partners in the development of our product such as an engineering team, manufacturing services, and regulatory specialists for FDA (Food and Drug Administration) approval. Protecting your intellectual property is important, so all startups should work with a team of lawyers. With our team of lawyers, we now have a utility patent for our technology. Our device was officially renamed Manoula, the Greek term of endearment for mothers. We are just getting started. We plan on developing our MVP prototype in early 2020, and bringing the product to market in 2023.

My practice as a bedside nurse provides daily examples of how helpful this device can be. Mothers hear my story and say, "I wish I had that device, my experience would have been so different." I always wanted to make a difference, to be able to change someone's life, and these steps have led me down the path to do so. I am a nurse, a CEO, a student, and an innovator.

As nurses, we sit at the forefront of changing patients' lives. Our intuitions and passions lead us on the pathway of innovating and improving the lives of others. We have the power—we've never been "just a nurse." Trust those gut instincts, act on pivotal feelings and inquiries, and follow these actions toward your goals. Like those before us, we are nurses, but most importantly, we are innovators.

SUPPLEMENTAL RESOURCES

- UCONN, the Healthcare Innovations Program
  https://cnsi.uconn.edu/healthcare-innovation
- Breastfeeding Statistics
  https://www.ncbi.nlm.nih.gov/books/NBK52687
  https://www.cdc.gov/breastfeeding/data/facts.html
- Patent search, market penetration, and the product's project revenue costs and regulatory pathway
  https://www.entrepreneur.com/article/196928
  https://www.educba.com/market-penetration
  https://www.fda.gov/patients/device-development-process/step-3-pathway-approval
  https://docs.oracle.com/cd/E41948_01/fscm92pbh1/eng/fscm/fprc/concept_Understanding ProjectCostandRevenueBudgets-9f3239.html
- LLC, Lactation Innovations
  www.lactationinnovations.com
- How to submit a grant for funding
  https://sbir.nih.gov
  https://sbir.nih.gov/funding
- Connecticut Children's Medical Center
  https://www.connecticutchildrens.org
- CEO/COO
  https://www.linkedin.com/pulse/difference-between-ceo-coo-jeyakumar-balasundararam

Becoming a "Nurse on Purpose"

CHINELO OFOMA, MSN, RN, CPNP-PC, FIEL

"WE AREN'T MERELY TRAINED IN PERFORMING CLINICAL SKILLS OR PROCEDURES—WE ARE PREPARED TO BE HEALTHCARE LEADERS, PUBLIC HEALTH CHAMPIONS, PUBLISHERS, POLICY INFLUENCERS, AND MUCH MORE."

Many have awe-inspiring stories of how they came into nursing; yet some of us simply felt drawn to it, following its bread trail until we finally felt that we were meant to be there. Nursing has been a deep calling and a dilemma. Despite a continuous inner conflict, a worthy purpose exists within my profession and I aim to attain it, all while struggling with the voices that so often urged me to choose a different, more "reputable" path.

I migrated to the United States after completing high school and choosing a career in accounting to follow in my mother's footsteps. In the developing world, nursing has been and continues to be a disregarded profession, so I never had the initial thought to pursue it. However, I was presented with the idea of a career in healthcare my sophomore year in college, and I began to explore the various options. Eventually, I chose nursing. Throughout my experiences in this profession, I am continuously reminded of my own special purpose within the grand scheme of healthcare.

To begin my journey, I had to apply as a transfer student into the nursing program, which everyone swore was an impossible feat. Many of the students who applied alongside me were not accepted and had to leave the school if they wanted to continue on their path to nursing. My acceptance was truly a gift. I was neither the most qualified nor the most deserving. Others applied to many other schools, just to have a safety net, but I didn't. I was gambling with the idea that if I didn't get in, then I would know that nursing was not for me.

People may be unaware of the depth of training that nurses receive or just how rigorous nursing programs are. We aren't merely trained in performing clinical skills or procedures—we are prepared to be healthcare leaders, public health champions, publishers, policy influencers, and much more.

During my time at Rutgers University, I had my eye on the prestigious University of Pennsylvania, where I would obtain my master's degree. I applied and, like before, did not apply to any other schools; rather, I put my best effort into one. Deep in my heart though, UPenn was a pipe dream, because, surely, I wasn't the kind of person to attend an Ivy League university. But I knew better than to give up on a dream without trying. When the acceptance letter came, I was stunned! The world was trying to tell me something that I had not quite grasped—when you are diligent, you become as capable and as worthy of success as anyone else.

While completing my master's studies, I worked full-time as an RN and commuted from New Jersey to Pennsylvania to attend school part-time. This period taught me a lot about my own resilience, especially during those last few highly demanding semesters. Being able to juggle the rigors of school with my work responsibilities really elevated my skill of focused time management, and to top it off, I graduated with high honors. Following graduation, I applied and went on to become one of two fellows selected among hundreds of applicants accepted into Carolinas Healthcare System's (now Atrium Health) fellowship cohort for Ambulatory Pediatrics in 2016—the largest nurse practitioner (NP) fellowship in the country with regard to the number of specialties and class size.

On the day of my interview, there were other highly qualified applicants, many from top universities, bearing experience and accomplishments I had not yet dreamed of. The interview went very well; again, self-doubt crept in—What were the odds of being selected? They were accepting two people from my specialty and hundreds applied. I decided that, if nothing else, I gave it my best shot after being lucky enough to be chosen for an interview. Not only was I accepted, my peers selected me to be the graduating speaker for my class at the end of the year-long program. A very high honor!

What do others see in you that you don't see in yourself? This is an invaluable question to ponder and inquire of those closest to you. Others can call out the greatness in you before you ever notice it in yourself.

The fellowship year consisted of clinical hours, didactic sessions, classroom presentations, and specialty rotations. With some initial preceptor oversight, fellows started out with very low daily patient volumes at our respective clinics. This gave us a chance to be as thorough as possible when seeing our patients, creating plans of care, looking up pertinent information, and deciding on the best treatment plans before presenting to our preceptor. As the weeks and months progressed, so did our patient volumes. Eventually, we were able to see as many patients as any provider in our clinic, and do so efficiently. The didactic sessions were student-led with a facilitator who was responsible for selecting our topics of discussion. Each fellow, on a rotational basis, was required to research the assigned topic and present to the group during our weekly sessions. There were corresponding discussion questions and we all had to be prepared for the week's topic, whether or not it was assigned to us. The topics were presented in the form of case studies and required critical thought processes in order to form our diagnoses and treatment modalities.

In addition, the fellows also had the chance to rotate through several specialty settings. For instance, as a Pediatric Fellow, I rotated through all things pediatrics, including pediatric gastroenterology, pediatric neurology, orthopedics, urology, hematology/oncology, surgery, pediatric urgent care, allergy and immunology, newborn nursery, endocrinology, dermatology, behavioral and developmental pediatrics, and so forth. Understanding several specialties gave me a great appreciation for their work and allowed me to teach my own patients with greater confidence regarding certain other diseases that are not typically seen in the primary care setting.

I was most proud of the fact that many of the clinicians I shadowed in these settings were nurse practitioners like myself, and they were extremely knowledgeable and skilled in their provision of care. They taught me so much, both clinically and professionally—their unwavering confidence and passion for nursing was admirable. The entire fellowship experience enhanced my drive to achieve more for our profession and my will to take risks that would propel us forward as a whole.

Even with each accomplishment, that fierce inner conflict to pursue a "more reputable" calling still existed. I have a deep desire to change the way the world views nurses: for others to see nursing as a highly respected and sought after profession at the forefront of healthcare innovation and healthcare policy decision-making. I was tired of hearing "oh you should have become a doctor," "you're too pretty to be just a nurse," "are you going to go to medical school after your NP degree?" Many popular TV shows continue to reinforce unflattering portrayals of nurses and underestimate the value of the work we do.

After my fellowship year, I decided to enter into the world of locum tenens to follow my passion for travel. As a locum pediatric nurse practitioner, I visit various cities and clinics providing primary care coverage as needed. This lifestyle provides the freedom to work on establishing my organization, Nurse On Purpose, which aims to challenge media stereotypes of nursing and pursue other callings, such as medical mission work.

Nurse On Purpose was born out of a passionate desire to create positive change in the world's perception of nurses. By challenging media stereotypes and calling nurses to professional and societal action, we support and spread the greater expression of a nurse's impact on their patients, their hospital, and their community. Nurses are intelligent, critical thinkers who make lifesaving decisions in their fields of practice. We are scientific researchers, patient advocates, and community leaders. Nurses at the master's and doctoral levels are able to diagnose, treat, and fully manage their patient's care. We are so often exposed to media images of the nurse standing around taking physician's orders; the unintelligent, unkempt, loud-mouthed nurse who treats patients with a lack of respect and patience; the unprofessional nurse who behaves inappropriately in the workplace; the "let me get the doctor for you" nurse who has no independent problem-solving skills; and so on.

It is the aim of Nurse On Purpose to continue to bring this awareness to mainstream media and address it in order to effect change. It must be understood that the reinforcement of these negative stereotypes is highly detrimental to the elevation of a profession as selfless as nursing, which has been long undervalued.

It took a long time to decide on a name for my organization. In fact, it took a long time to even begin creating an organization, for fear of launching and falling flat on my face. But I was frustrated enough, and I figured that I could either dare to make a difference or could continue to endure in silence. I finally started at the end of 2018. As I established myself on social networking platforms, I received positive feedback and formed professional connections. A single bold step has led to many open doors and opportunities.

Launch and give yourself permission to fall as many times as it takes, or you may always regret not having tried.

Being a part of SONSIEL means that I join a community of nurse innovators, business owners, dreamers, thinkers, and doers who are not afraid to push the envelope; nurses who want better for our profession and are striving to create it. I realize now that the conflict existed because there was work to be done. Opting for something different would mean taking the easy way out—however, as it is said—"no guts, no glory."

My story is far from over, but to share the initial parts of it in this book is an honor. When others read it, my hope is that they also feel the courage to step out in faith, answer the deep call within, and use what they've been gifted with.

SUPPLEMENTAL RESOURCES

- Carolinas Healthcare System's (now Atrium Health) fellowship cohort for Ambulatory Pediatrics
  https://atriumhealth.org/education/center-for-advanced-practice/fellowships
- Nurse On Purpose
  http://www.nurseonpurpose.org
- An article on media stereotypes of nurses
  http://www.nursing.columbia.edu/nurses-media
- An article or resource on how to use social media to launch an organization
  http://ojin.nursingworld.org/MainMenuCategories/ANAMarketplace/ANAPeriodicals/OJIN/TableofContents/Vol-19-2014/No3-Sept-2014/Insights-for-Promoting-Health.html

Nothing Motivates You More Than the Fear of Losing It All

WENDY WRIGHT, DNP, ANP-BC, FNP-BC, FAANP, FAAN, FNAP

"As a nurse practitioner, I had counseled patients regularly about finding a job they loved. I needed to heed my own counsel."

In late 2006, I noticed that I was waking up every Monday dreading the prospect of having to go to my job. Yes, I called it a job because somehow over the past few years, my work had become just that. I was working as a family nurse practitioner in an MD-owned family practice in southern New Hampshire. The physician and I had worked together for the past 11 years. I had always loved my work, until recently. I had grown my panel to more than 1,000 patients, carved out my place in the clinic with a group of devoted patients, and had a job-share partner who was truly the best. However, the clinic environment was rapidly becoming a place of discontent. We (the nurse practitioners [NPs]) were being asked to see more patients, return more calls, handle more tasks, and yet, there was never any discussion of pay raises or additional benefits. Previously devoted to providing the best practices of healthcare, this environment became something that I no longer recognized and a place that I could no longer work. I was heartbroken. I truly envisioned myself finishing my career alongside this physician. Yet, patient care was being compromised and I could no longer willingly be part of it. As a nurse practitioner, I had counseled patients regularly about finding a job they loved. I needed to heed my own counsel.

After much thought, I resigned my clinical practice in December 2006, truly having no idea what the next 30 years of my career would look like. I planned on taking some time to write, teach, be a mom, and just figure it out. But that was not in the cards. During a vacation with my sister, who had just opened a surgical center for a group of urologists, she suggested that we open a family practice together. Of course, I would be responsible for paying for the clinic (I am the older sister) but she would do the set-up and be instrumental in the opening. We would bring along a part-time NP—my job-share partner who was planning on leaving the clinic when I did—and a billing/practice manager to assist with the start-up. It took a week of her unrelenting nagging for me to consent, but I took the proverbial leap. In the next 6 weeks, I mortgaged my home, found an office building, and set up a full-service family practice. Opening a full-service clinic in 6 weeks is a herculean task. Everything from finding rental space, ordering supplies, credentialing with insurance companies, contracting with suppliers and an electronic health system, and marketing had to be conducted in this 6-week period. These tasks usually take a well-oiled hospital system more than 6 months. Yet, our team of three did it in 6 weeks. We worked around the clock, each taking shifts. We called on friends and family to clean, paint, market the clinic door-to-door, and call vendors. They say it takes a village and I couldn't agree more.

We opened on February 1, 2007, with seven patients on the books and another 90 or so who had called to voice their intent to join. Within 6 months, the practice had grown to 500 patients. By one year, we were at 1,000 patients. I was fortunate to have a speaking career already established, so I was able to put every bit of income from the clinic, back into the clinic to pay off all debt and expand the services. By month 6, all start-up costs were paid, including the loan on my home. Today, this clinic has approximately 4,500 patients and six NPs. In 2012, I opened a second clinic located in Concord, New Hampshire. I knew that

Concord would be a perfect area as there were no primary care providers taking on any new patients at the time. This clinic has grown to 2,000 patients and is staffed by three full-time NPs. We generally hire NPs who have been students within the clinic. We have found that it gives them an opportunity to assess us while giving us a chance to see if we will be a good fit for them. Today, my sister Becky is the practice manager in both businesses.

The primary care clinics are not like many you will find. First and foremost, they are owned and operated by NPs and medical assistants (MAs) only. Each person works to the upper limit of her education and training. Second, each visit is a minimum of 30 minutes, with many visits booked for 45 to 60 minutes. Patients are afforded time to discuss their concerns and the NPs are given time to discuss theirs. The NPs average 10 to 12 patient visits per day. All new graduate NPs are offered a 2-year mentorship where they are given a graduated patient schedule and have their charts reviewed nightly, all while receiving full pay. A lead NP is available every day in the clinics to provide guidance and consultations, if needed. The NPs have quarterly meetings with the lead NP to discuss concerns, discuss new guidelines, and propose clinic changes. Each patient visit is pre-visit care-planned by an MA who has been trained in national guidelines. For instance, every patient's chart is reviewed prior to the visit to determine the need for recommended screening tests and vaccinations. NPs are provided with this information to ensure that the recommended preventive services are offered to every patient at every visit.

The providers and staff have won numerous awards for their work, including the 2018 Top Family Practice Providers in Souhegan Valley, New Hampshire. This is the first time an NP-owned clinic has received this award. We have also been listed in the Top 20 Fastest Growing Family Business and Top 20 Women-Owned Businesses in New Hampshire by *Business Review* magazine of NH. As a result of the success of our clinics and the excellence of our employees, I received the 2014 Top 5 Women in New Hampshire Business Award.

We are currently growing at a rate of more than 100 new patients per month without any formal advertising. The reputation of the providers and staff within the community has made our clinics a go-to source for patients looking for primary care providers. Over the past 2 years, we have partnered with two drug-treatment facilities to provide comprehensive primary care services to patients with substance use disorders. We are proud of the work we have done to ensure these individuals get rapid, personalized, and compassionate primary care within days of discharge from the treatment facilities. We also offer numerous point-of-care tests and services including home sleep studies, pulmonary function testing, lesion biopsies, laceration repair, and acute and chronic disease management. In addition, we rent space to physical therapy and a full-service national lab. These onsite services minimize the need for patients to travel to other venues and improve the likelihood of treatment adherence.

In 2013, Blue Cross/Blue Shield of NH, along with the NP practice owners of NH, formed the first accountable care organization (ACO) in the nation made up of NP-managed patients. Data from this novel ACO provided evidence that NP-managed patients have equal quality metric scores to those of our physician colleagues, have some of the lowest hospital admission rates in the state, and cost the insurer approximately $60.00 less per month than MD-managed patients. In fact, a few of the NP clinics have some of the highest quality metric scores in the state of NH. Data from this project were published by this author in the January 2016 edition of *Nursing Administration Quarterly*.

In addition to our ACO work, Wright & Associates Family Healthcare @Amherst and @Concord have partnered with two local universities, their faculty, and their master's and doctoral NP students to make our sites and clinical data available for the students to use for Capstone and quality improvement projects. The students develop the projects, collect data, present summaries of current clinical care, and based upon the results, present recommendations for quality improvement. Results from each project are published in a national NP journal by the students, faculty, and this author. Through these annual partnerships, care is improved for our patients without expending significant fiscal resources.

Today, our annual billables for the two clinics are in excess of $3 million, with an annual payroll of more than $1.2 million. All staff, including MAs and NPs, receive annual peer reviews and pay increases, if earned. We pay 100% of every employee's health, vision, and dental insurances. While we expect a lot from every employee on staff, we also recognize that a healthy employee comes from a healthy workplace. Each employee begins with a minimum of 3 weeks of earned time plus eight to 11 holidays annually. We do quarterly outings/events for the staff such as baseball nights, pool parties, holiday parties, and wine tastings to reward the staff for their dedication. When the company is financially able, annual bonuses are given to each employee based upon the years of employment.

These clinics have become training sites for NPs around the nation interested in business ownership. NPs can spend a day or a week with the management and staff to be mentored in business ownership. In addition, the practice manager and owner conduct quarterly meetings for all NP business owners in the state to address local, state, and national issues that may affect practice. These meetings have been running for 13 years and are attended by more than 20 NP business owners.

While these clinics have been very successful, I have made numerous mistakes throughout the course of my business career. My reasons for writing this story is to show you that anything is possible with a little hard work, but also to help you avoid the mistakes I have made.

I grew up in a trailer park in rural NH. I was raised by two amazing parents, neither of whom graduated high school. Both of my parents, however, had a work ethic that surpassed most. They taught us that nothing is impossible if you are willing to work hard. Running these clinics is by far the hardest work I have ever done, but it is also great to see the fruits of our labor and to celebrate our successes.

My best advice to anyone wanting to innovate is:

- Make sure you are ready to work 7 days per week for years to get your business up and running and running well.

- Start low and go slow—don't hire people that you don't need. Ramp up as you go.

- Surround yourself with people who share the same vision as you.

- Reward your staff; they are your best assets.

- The first time you think about firing someone, do it! Hire slowly, fire quickly! Bad employees can quickly ruin all you have worked to build.

- Not everyone is your friend. It's okay. A business needs a leader not a friend.

- Take the leap—it is worth it!

SUPPLEMENTAL RESOURCES

- *Nurse Practitioner's Business Practice and Legal Guide*, 4th ed.
  https://www.amazon.com/Nurse-Practitioners-Business-Practice-Legal/dp/B006RVF39E
- *NH Business Review* Magazine
  https://www.nhbr.com/
- The Best of Business (BOB) Awards
  https://www.nhbr.com/events-awards/best-of-business-awards/

- The Outstanding Women in Business Awards
  nhbr.com/events-awards/outstanding-women-in-business/
- Wright & Associates Family Healthcare
  https://wrightfhc.com/
- *Nurse-Led Health Clinics: Operations, Policy, and Opportunities*
  https://www.springerpub.com/nurse-led-health-clinics-9780826128027.html
- *Economics and Financial Management for Nurses and Nurse Leaders*, 3rd ed.
  https://www.springerpub.com/economics-and-financial-management-for-nurses-and-nurse-leaders-third-edition-9780826160010.html

I Am a Nurse

JOAN GURVIS SHIELDS, MSN, RN

"*OUR BRAINS DEFINED US, NOT THE TRADITION.*"

There it was again. The choice point, filled with that familiar hesitation, an unwillingness to reveal the shame that sometimes followed the withholding. Why, I asked myself, was it so hard to roll the words over my tongue and say with confidence, "I am a nurse."

My career has taken so many wonderful and unexpected turns such that I now stand in front of CEOs and senior leaders from all around the world on a very regular basis. Those from every industry, representing Fortune 50 and 100 companies, are all asking for my help. How did I get here, you might wonder: a senior faculty member with the Center for Creative Leadership (CCL; a global nonprofit provider of Executive Education) and former Managing Director of CCL Colorado Springs Business Unit?

I suppose you could say it started when my father was diagnosed with polycystic kidney disease at a time when dialysis was only provided to the very few patients who "would live." He was accepted into a government-sponsored program and remained on dialysis for over 20 years—despite one kidney rupture later and multiple other debilitating side effects. I watched my mother care for him while they both held down full-time jobs. They had my sister and me to put through college, the first generation of children in their families to have that opportunity. We were the daughters of two blue collar workers—a telephone repairman and a school secretary. I learned to sit with him and study while he was having treatments, watching the nurses expertly manage their patients who depended upon them: the tricks they had for hypotension after a dialysis run, how to make the extremely low sodium diet taste a bit more palatable, and being an ongoing witness to their lives. When my father passed away 25 years later, the funeral home was filled with visitors. I was visibly shaken when I learned how much they knew about my father—a man of few words—and how embedded he was in their hearts. I knew I wanted to be like him.

Or, it could have been in 1970, when my best friend, Laurie Carr, and I were freshmen in high school. We watched our friends' older brothers and my sister go off to some place in Asia called Vietnam and never come home. We vowed we would become Navy nurses and do it the quickest way possible, by attending a diploma school of nursing. In a few short years after graduation, we would be on the field somewhere holding the hands of wounded or dying soldiers—making a difference, alleviating their suffering.

To make my parents happy, I did apply to 4-year colleges and my fail-safe opportunity was the New England Deaconess School of Nursing. Off my mother and I went to Boston to meet with the dean, a lovely woman with her hair in a French twist. Very professional, direct, and kind. She looked at me with her piercing blue eyes and said, "I am accepting you on the spot and also rejecting you." My head was spinning. She went on to say to me, "You are in the top 20 in your high school class of 325 and your SAT scores are outstanding. The future of nursing is at the baccalaureate level. You need to bypass your diploma and go for your BSN. Best wishes." I wish I could remember her name, as I think of that day often and how it changed my life.

It was March and I was in a bit of a dilemma. I had not really put much thought into my college picks. I was conscious of my family's limited finances. My mother pushed me to look harder. I browsed through the college catalogues and found the one, Duke University. I stayed up for two nights filling out the application packet. The month of May brought a rejection letter. What now? After quite some time, the secretary called, "I am so sorry, we sent you the wrong letter; you have been accepted into the Class of 77 School of Nursing." With a handful of loans and one suitcase, I showed up in August sight unseen at one of the most prestigious universities in the country.

My life at Duke fundamentally changed me as a person. In my freshman *Intro to Nursing* lecture course, Dr. Pauline Graatz pointed her finger at us and said with fierce conviction, "You are the best and the brightest. You are the future of nursing. Be leaders, be researchers, be the best practitioners you can be, but above all, you must change the future of nursing." Between Dr. Graatz and Dean Ruby Wilson, there was no room to question their charge. So, we went off into the world, my peers and I, to become nurse practitioners, nurse administrators, entrepreneurs, attorneys, clinical experts, chief operating officers, CEOs, and business leaders. Three years ago at my Duke reunion, Dr. Wilson was there in a wheelchair. She remembered most of us. When she saw me she asked, "Well, did you do it? Did you make good on your word to change the future of nursing?" I felt lost in my response. What had I done really with that charge?

After graduating from Duke, I held a variety of clinical roles specializing in critical care— open heart and cardiovascular surgery/trauma. At the tender age of 21, I was the night charge nurse in a 22-bed surgical ICU in Columbus, Ohio. I struggled with managing my patient load, learning all the machines and technology. Duke did not exactly prepare us to care for "ordinary patients." Yet, they taught me how to think on my feet, to watch and observe intently, to believe in myself, and not to fall into being a handmaiden. I was written up for not wearing my nursing cap on a few occasions. Why would I put a coffee filter on my head in place of a cap? We never wore them at Duke, so why start now? Our brains defined us, not the tradition.

I worked in the cardiac catheterization lab at Miami Heart Institute, assisting with the very first angioplasty and conduction studies. I was determined to gain my critical care (CCRN) certification and studied day and night for 6 months. I was so proud to be conferred that certification, passing with high marks. I learned that I love teaching others, so I became a clinical preceptor and then a nurse educator. From that, I moved into an organizational development practice at a large teaching hospital in Florida working with nurse leaders and hospital administrators, helping them to navigate the waves of change, then headed to graduate school for an MSN. I was unsuccessful in designing a combo graduate degree with business administration

(MSN-MBA). The dual degree was created a year after I graduated. More certifications and a graduate degree later, I was asked to lead a nurse intern program in a large teaching hospital in North Carolina. I began speaking and writing on competency-based education and soon founded a small consulting business as an expert witness for nursing practice. Yet I felt stuck, ineffective, and unable to inoculate change. Burnt out and tired, I fled healthcare. With a short stop at a wealth management company, I arrived at the Center for Creative Leadership. Hired as a faculty member for my business savvy, I was rapidly promoted to senior management and led the Greensboro, NC, and then Colorado Springs, CO, campus' multimillion dollar business units.

"How did you make the transition from nursing," people would always ask once they found out I was a nurse, as I facilitated their leadership development experiences. "I never really left." I use the nursing process every day in the business world. It helps me to observe people, to understand the nuances of human behavior, to rely on evidence-based practices, to think on my feet, and to integrate differing perspectives. Nursing allows me to be a better leader, executive coach, and leadership facilitator.

At CCL, I have had the privilege of working with many health and healthcare executives building high performing teams, driving culture change, and coaching senior leaders. One of my most rewarding assignments was designing the Robert Wood Johnson Foundation (RWJF) *Executive Nurse Fellows* Program from 2006 until 2018 with other CCL colleagues. The talent of those Fellows in the room blew me away. If only I had known where my career could have taken me in nursing. Suddenly, I did not have a nursing mentor; someone to guide me along, to inspire and challenge me to do more—to light the way. I was creating an entirely uncharted path for myself.

I am so proud of where I am today, especially knowing the impact I make and the lives I touch—albeit in a different way—is still making a difference. Because, I also now know the experience of sitting across from a leader, holding the space between us in conversation, assessing and observing, forming a hypothesis, planning a way forward, executing, and evaluating. In the end, I suppose it is fair to say I practice nursing, but in a different way. I never really left. My path was different.

I have been deeply honored to share my story in this book, and humbled by the company it keeps. As a nurse, you have unlimited possibilities. You are a master of humanity. No matter where your journey takes you, my hope is that you will always find your voice and be able to say with certainty and without hesitation, "I am a nurse." My hope is also that you will never second-guess your value or worry about what others will think of you. You have earned your right to a seat at the table. Seize the moment and be the best you can be.

SUPPLEMENTAL RESOURCES

- Center for Creative Leadership
  https://www.ccl.org
- Duke University, School of Nursing
  https://nursing.duke.edu
- CCRN certification
  https://www.aacn.org/certification/get-certified/ccrn-adult
- Adult CCRN Certification Review: Think in Questions, Learn by Rationale
  https://www.springerpub.com/adult-ccrn-certification-review-9780826198334.html
- Robert Wood Johnson Foundation (RWJF) *Executive Nurse Fellows* Program
  https://www.nursetrust.org

The Rebel Nurse's Progress Note

We hope these stories have allowed you to recognize the incredible opportunity you have to uniquely transform the health of others. Consider and be willing to advocate and use your voice. Through mentorship and following the success of others that have led the way, you are able to gain the courage you need to advocate for yourself and for others. It is usually the mentors and the other supporters in our lives who help to call out the greatness in us before we even realize it in ourselves. And as many have shared, you must be willing to leverage that trust to advocate for others.

Choose to see nursing as an art and as a science, acknowledging that the opportunity to teach and make a difference for future generations may be at the bedside, as well as beyond. Choose to be great at what you're good at and continue to push yourself past comfort. Although failure may feel inevitable, be willing to overcome your fears.

Throughout your journey to gaining the boldness and confidence you need to embrace the *rebel nurse* that you are, be willing to ask yourself, "What would you do if you couldn't fail?" And even if you do fail, keep trying anyway. There are always ways to be creative, as long as you're willing to search for new opportunities.

As *rebel nurses*, we should realize that this journey to become a shift disruptor constitutes refusing to be put in a box or limited, whether by others or yourself. Sometimes you may have to challenge media stereotypes or take a professional or societal stance on an issue, you may have to work around the clock in the beginning, and you may have to recognize early on that not everyone is your "friend." This idea is not always easy to hear, but an important one to consider when choosing to make big change. As long as you're willing to trust your gut instincts, even when life is not easy, even in the face of rejection, you can take hold of life's most pivotal moments and shift them in your favor.

Always be willing to meet someone new or to learn something new. Consider networking to form relationships, especially ones that help you push the boundaries of your comfort zone. Learn, early on, how to protect your intellectual property as you embrace innovation; or even how to build pitch decks for an invention. Whatever the case, as you learn, be willing to allow your vision to inspire your path, as well as embrace life's trials, rather than run from them.

And, most importantly, know that in all things, nurses work with humanity. It is in that humanity that you, as a nurse, may find your voice, and speak boldly about being the *rebel nurse* that you are. You were designed and destined for greatness.

{ *Where in your career are you willing to disrupt the status quo? How did these stories motivate you to action?* }

Overcoming the Odds: Pioneer Nurses Blazing Trails Around the World

To be resilient is to stand strong when it seems everything should knock you down. It is the ability to withstand the challenges of life, maybe not unscathed, but with the perspective to see how your own story or journey can change the life of another. These nurses, these trailblazers, these pioneers defied the odds—financial hardships, unimaginable family expectations and responsibilities, health and medical limitations, and societal pushback—and dared to go beyond the seeming limitations of life to change their sphere of influence. These nurses have paid the price and it shows proudly throughout the prestigious influence they have on healthcare.

A Nurse's Diagnoses

RICHARD MOORE, PhD, DPROF(c), MBA, MSc (CARDIOLOGY), BSc (HONS), RN, RNT, DMS, FIMGT, FHEA, FESC, FIEL, FRSPH, JP

"IT IS AN UTTER PRIVILEGE BEING A REGISTERED NURSE WHO WORKS ALONGSIDE NURSES WHO MOVE THE BOUNDARIES OF EXCELLENCE—THAT RAREFIED CLINICIAN ORBITING THE HIGHEST ALTITUDES OF PROFESSIONAL BRILLIANCE."

"Don't eat anything at this place if you're offered food," my mom spoke as we turned the corner into a drive full of weeds, overgrown bushes, and a dilapidated, unkempt house. I was with her again on her house calls. My mom was a district nurse, later a district nursing officer, visiting clients in areas of the very poor and the very rich with their million-dollar houses. Even though I was 7 years old, I was already a veteran of diplomacy with people—quietness, observing, listening, and following mom. Some of her clients had no wooden floors, because they had used them for firewood to keep warm, and they kept their babies in open drawers. You had to take care of where you walked.

I had no options. My dad died when I was 9 days old at Obuasi gold mine, Ghana, and my sister, 11 years old, had left home. It was simply mom and I. In my 5 years of high school, my grades were so poor. I became the only student to finish in last place every year that I attended. It wasn't looking good for the future. I left school at 16 to follow my mom and sister into nursing. Nursing was the only thing I knew.

With private tuition, I gained just enough qualifications to enter nursing. But the stakes were so high. My mom, sister, and aunt had all been educated at St. James's University Hospital, Leeds, Europe's largest teaching hospital. Set on 50 acres with 1,157 beds, it was a village, not a hospital. Its education of nurses was renowned as world class. In our family, this was the only place to apply. It could not be anywhere else. Thankfully, I was accepted—but would I survive? Survive living in the nurse's home of 400 students? Survive the education and assessments? Would I enjoy nursing at all? It was one thing going around with mom for years, another to actually be a nurse.

I needn't have worried. I loved nursing—the hospital, the friends I made, the joie de vivre. But in my second year, while on my pediatric placement, disaster struck. I was diagnosed with ulcerative colitis. I had been passing blood for a few days with increasing urgency and motions. I saw a gastroenterologist, had a colonoscopy, and started azathioprine, an immunosuppressant. With relapses and remissions throughout, I managed to complete my nurse education and register as an RN. Through this storm, I realized that I have heaps to offer in making a difference in nursing. I could use this experience to help others. So I set out to get the best education possible, learn from other brilliant clinicians, and ultimately make a difference. That meant thinking laterally, innovatively, and changing systems.

My questions changed: What's my aim? Where am I going here? What do I want to do? I was offered five jobs. I had a real interest in all things heart, so I planned to manage a ward first, gaining clinical management expertise, then work in ICU with the sickest patients. I would finally be ready for the cardiac care unit (CCU), combining both skills. So that's what I did. I completed orthopedics, ICU, and CCU.

I loved and continue to love the CCU. The combination of quiet, patient interaction, giving rehabilitation advice to cardiac arrests, EKG interpretation and rhythm analysis, and so much more. I found my clinical home. I applied and became a charge nurse in CCU, a job I loved. It was then that I had to plan. Do I head to education or management? I loved both. I completed a postgraduate diploma in management studies, and during this time, I had changed the CCU procurement system to align with real-time budgets and stock control. Senior management rewarded my work by asking me to join a hospital-wide project with Lucas Systems and Engineering. I was very humbled. I was simply doing my job.

The project focused on procurement with the belief that savings could be gained while improving the systems. I grew skills as a management consultant, using critical thinking skills to understand how systems worked. This knowledge was also beneficial for completing my MBA. It was also useful for implementing ISO 9001 within a friend's law firm, making them one of the first in the United Kingdom to have a quality benchmark. I was offered a senior manager's job, an assistant chief nurse rank, to continue the project's board-approved recommendations. I was 26.

It took a team to revolutionize procurement across this monster of a hospital. We saved millions of pounds of public money, recurring almost every year, and built systems to ensure every part of procurement was world class. We studied Toyota's world-class procurement system and adapted it to a hospital setting. New products were researched before anyone even thought about purchasing them. The stock was driven down to 2 weeks of supply across the board. On every ward and unit, electronic data interchanges were established with every product quantity, price, and location known. The work was extremely revolutionary in the early 1990s.

After 3 years, I decided to leave and follow my other passion—education. I started commuting to London, 220 miles away, to become a casual lecturer at Thames Valley University. I'd stay a few days and return home. I was quickly given the University's English National Board 124 Coronary Care Program to look after. Fourteen London hospitals sent their staff on this postgraduate program to become experts in coronary care nursing. I was attached to the Circulatory Sciences directorate at St. Mary's Hospital, Paddington, as an honorary senior lecturer and formulated the United Kingdom's first nurse-led postgraduate thrombolysis program that gained university and regulatory approval. I moved to arguably the most prestigious nursing school in London, the Florence Nightingale School of Nursing at King's College, University of London; started living in London; and qualified as a fellow of the higher education academy. I was appointed a senior lecturer back at Thames Valley University and acting director of standards at arguably the National Health Service's flagship hospital, Chelsea and Westminster Hospital, a little later. I was 32.

I then took a year off to travel around the world, primarily to find a home to emigrate to. I'd known for some time the United Kingdom was not my place to live and, with faith, left the United Kingdom to visit Singapore, Australia, New Zealand, Cook Islands, and the United States. I emigrated to New Zealand, and was offered a senior academic staff member job at Eastern Institute of Technology primarily to coordinate the master's level multidisciplinary health service management program.

I loved New Zealand and worked at the Eastern Institute of Technology. During my tenure, I was humbled with extraordinary opportunities. I directed the master of nursing degree and postgraduate programs. I was asked by the district health board chief executive to lead a team to ensure fiscal sustainability from an $8 million debt. I formulated New Zealand's first master's level postgraduate coronary and intensive care program for nurses that received full regulatory approval.

After 5 years, I had a strong sense to leave, so in faith, I did. I had no job, but the decision was correct. After a few months, I found myself in the Tanami Desert in the Northern Territory,

Australia. I was a remote area nurse looking after the Warlpiri people providing every conceivable healthcare from acute trauma to primary health for children to adults. I felt stretched, exhilarated, and sheer stunned at times. The breadth and depth of the role were vast. I was on call through the night for all emergencies, including cannulating sick dogs with acute on chronic renal failure. There are no vets. I worked with only two other nurses. The longest I worked straight was a perfect storm of a remote area, raining so the plane couldn't land on the sand runway, and two critically ill patients arriving together; one with acute pancreatitis, the other with an anterior ST-segment elevation myocardial infarction (STEMI). It was 30 hours nonstop work, finally finishing when the Royal Doctors Flying Service (RFDS) plane landed with the retrieval RFDS nurse giving us a bar of chocolate as they'd heard about us flagging!

I commuted from New Zealand to Australia for 2 years as a remote area nurse and became aware of a side of nursing I'd never seen, let alone managed, and was often alone. From a machete in a skull, to a diabetic coma 90 km across the desert from Uluru, to a full leg severed by a steel fence post to the bone, to babies with acute bronchiectasis, to acute psychosis, to vaccinations. I loved it: the outback, the nursing, the people, and the deserts.

After emigrating across the ditch to Australia, I was asked by health executives to direct hospitals in the outback. These remote hospitals serve as the only health facility in an area sometimes the size of a million square kilometers. My previous experience of a remote area nurse and management helped enormously. I still nursed patients, too, particularly patients with cardiology problems. Working in the remote outback presented very different challenges. "Who is in the zoo?" is a question all remote area nurses ask. It means, "Who's in the team, and what client based do we have?" *Do we have a midwife? Who's good with mental health patients? If we have a STEMI, who's the best?* You work closely with people, and innovation is vital. You see, as the director of nursing here, you're not just the boss or an RN. You're the staff counselor, the landlord for health property, the face of health to the elders and native title holders, the generator checker, chemical expert, public health "physician," primary health advisor to the local council, chief police liaison officer, hotel manager for accommodating visiting health clinicians, and director of major incidents, to name a few. I dealt with a plane crash and category 5 cyclones. Oh, and chief toilet sorter-outer, too!

During this time, I was humbled again. I was asked by the health service chief executive to work alongside Methven Consulting to ensure long-term fiscal sustainability as a result of government budget cuts, and further as project director undertaking the director-general-mandated business planning framework across Cape York. The latter reviewed all nursing roles, occasions of service, and budgets. I finally was awarded a fellow of the European Society of Cardiology.

It was during this time when my son was around 6 years old that I noticed something. He altered during writing, dropping his pens, and could not concentrate. I thought he had dyscalculia. After a review by the director of pediatrics, they diagnosed Joshua with Asperger syndrome (now autistic spectrum disorder), attention deficit hyperactivity disorder (ADHD), and later auditory processing disorder. It was a relief, but then it hit. How on earth do we manage this? What's the best way forward? We read, researched, and chatted to people we trusted. It took me over a year to fully adjust to this and have a clear direction.

As I was researching, I noticed that many of the aspects, signs and symptoms, behaviors, and sensitivities were staring at me. It was both a bombshell and utter relief. I had struggled throughout all my life with many, many things. Seeing new people, talking to strangers, spelling, grammar, bright lights, sounds, learning by algorithms and visuals, focused on particular things, repetitive behavior, distractibility, and so on. A psychiatrist diagnosed me with Asperger syndrome (now autistic spectrum disorder), ADHD, and sensory processing disorder. I was given a new life.

Unfortunately, this wasn't the last diagnosis. I had noticed my brain function wasn't flowing as usual. It wasn't operating at its usual light speed. I couldn't keep up with people's conversations. I couldn't recall things, sometimes taking 30 seconds to be able to speak it out. And this was just the start. I think I blew several circuits in my brain overusing it. It was used to high volume, but not multiple layers of serious issues over a marathon run. It had run out of juice. I had severe clinical depression. I wanted to stay in bed, not see anyone, and not leave home. At times my brain couldn't function. It merely stopped, and I couldn't process a question, let alone answer it.

The psychiatrist I had seen previously, started treating me. Over 2 years, I recovered. I learned a lot of lessons and now have more wisdom about how I use my brain. One of those things I agreed was to enter the Hermit Kingdom, North Korea, as an adjunct professor within the School of Medicine and adjunct professor within their School of International Finance and Management. I was again very humbled, being the only RN within any North Korean university teaching medical students, doctors, and economists, too.

Throughout my career, I held fiercely to one thing—being an RN who maintains the craft, art, and science of nursing. Nursing is my role—an RN. Staff recognize that I walk their talk. Students know I take patient loads. Executives know I understand how to truly work under pressure. To me, it's crucial. It is an utter privilege being an RN who works alongside nurses who move the boundaries of excellence—that rarefied clinician, orbiting the highest altitudes of professional brilliance.

Nursing is a brilliant role. We make a difference for many people, often those who we don't know. If I—with my ulcerative colitis, autistic spectrum disorder, ADHD, sensory processing disorder, depression, coming last in high school, living in several countries, deserts, and rainforests—can nurse well, so can you. You can make a difference to patients, families, and staff. Every person is unique and has their own story. Find it and walk with them.

SUPPLEMENTAL RESOURCES

- St. James's University Hospital, Leeds
  https://www.leedsth.nhs.uk/patients-visitors/our-hospitals/st-james-university-hospital
- Thames Valley University
  https://www.uwl.ac.uk
- St. Mary's Hospital, Paddington
  https://www.imperial.nhs.uk/our-locations/st-marys-hospital
- Florence Nightingale School of Nursing at King's College, University of London
  https://www.kcl.ac.uk/nmpc
- Eastern Institute of Technology
  https://www.eit.ac.nz/subject-areas/health-professions
- Health Service Management Program
  https://www.eit.ac.nz/wp-content/uploads/programme-app-packs/Master%20of%20Nursing%20Science%202019,%20full%20pack%20PRINT%20READY.Pdf
- Methven Consulting
  http://www.echelongroup.co.nz

Why Did You Become a Nurse?

JALIL JOHNSON, PHD, MS, APRN, ANP-BC

"CREATE POSITIVE CHANGE THROUGH EMPOWERMENT AND ANY MEANS NECESSARY."

Why did you become a nurse? As an African American man in a female-dominated profession, people ask me this question often. The truth is, I started my healthcare career unintentionally.

I grew up the oldest of eight children, in a family that survived on an annual income of less than $10,000 in the rural South. To say my parents were all consumed with just keeping our family afloat would be an understatement. Perhaps they thought I was bright enough, or maybe they thought their token child would figure life out; regardless, I had no guidance. After I graduated high school, I set off into the world without a real plan. I had a partner. We were young, and not long after we started our relationship, I found myself to be a 19-year-old father of a baby girl. Throughout my life, my father always had trouble holding down a steady job. I was raised in abject poverty and as a new father, I promised myself I would never raise a family in that kind of despair.

I worked as many odd jobs as I could—assembly lines in warehouses, landfills, cutting tobacco, laying sod, security guards, and cleaning bathrooms in office buildings. Honestly, I didn't mind the work as long as I could provide for my family. The job that changed my life was the one I lost, as in, I was fired. I was working at a restaurant chain as a dishwasher. The work was dirty, but honest. I seemed to be treated fair for the most part, and it paid nearly $7.00/hour! Score!

One fateful evening, I stood in line at the time clock with four other employees, waiting to clock in. The shift manager approached, pointed to each and every one of us, and said in a dry, matter-of-fact kind of way, "You, you, you, and you. Y'all can go home."

As the other three started walking away, I asked, "I'll be back tomorrow, okay?"

She responded flatly, "Nah, you don't ever have to come back, I don't need ya."

I stayed and pleaded with her to allow me to stay and work or at least be allowed to come back the next day. I literally begged her. The manager shrugged her shoulders, lit a cigarette, and blew smoke in my face. She gave me a final warning, "You need to leave now … I don't need ya."

I caught the bus home. I was living check to check and now there was no check coming. The next day, I used some of the last remaining dollars I had to buy a box of Ramen noodles, some diapers, and a few cans of tuna. I spent the next few days looking for work, but kept coming up short. I was despondent, to say the least. On the third day, I kissed my baby goodbye, told her mother I was leaving, and wouldn't be back until I'd figured out how we were going to survive. I gave her five of my last 10 dollars and left our apartment, truly unsure of where to go or what to do.

I caught the bus to an area of the city where there were lots of restaurants and strip malls. I filled out applications all day and into the evening. When night came, I was too far from home to walk back and I only had $1.75 left in my pocket. I took a newspaper that was left on a table in the waffle house I'd applied to, and I decided to walk through the night for as long as my legs would carry me. When the street lights would allow enough light, I read the job section. There was an ad for free certified nursing assistant (CNA) classes at a local technical school on the other side of town. I walked through the night and slept for a few hours at the back of the school.

I spent the morning and afternoon applying for jobs near the school and at the school. That same evening, I asked the person at the information desk about the CNA program. Great news, the 4-week training was nearly FREE, but there was a catch. I needed to pay for the books. I had no money for books and the class was starting the next week.

It seemed like a hopeless situation. I left the information booth and sat on a bench in front of the school. The answer to my problems seemed so close ... but the roadblocks seemed unrelenting. I was determined to figure out how to make this work. As I sat pondering my next move, a man approached me. I must have looked pretty rough—hair in dreads, baggy pants, a thin frame, likely a bit dirty and smelly, and a scowl on my face. He asked, "How are you doing? Everything okay?"

I don't know why, but all my struggles poured out to this man. I told him about my job, my family, that I hadn't really slept last night, that I was hungry. I told him I just wanted to work. He *listened*.

Then he pulled out some cash and handed it to me. He said to come back tomorrow and ask to speak to Dr. King. I left the school with $17.75 in my pocket and a lot of uncertainty.

The next morning, I returned to the school and asked for Dr. King. That generous man was the dean of the school. He walked me over to the financial aid office and asked them to help me complete my financial aid package, emphasizing my need to start in the upcoming CNA course.

Dr. King didn't mention to anyone how he helped me out. In fact, he never mentioned it again. I remember thinking—*if I ever make it, I'm going to help people out the way he helped me*.

The next week I met my CNA instructor, Ms. Lewis. Ms. Lewis was a LPN and had worked in the local community hospital ED for over 20 years, until they started phasing out LPNs. Ms. Lewis approached teaching with true gusto—energetic, firm, and kind. In high school, teachers and course work were simply throughways to what I really wanted to do. To me, as an adult learner, Ms. Lewis was the first teacher who engaged me in a way that made me feel like I belonged in the room. After my first day of classes with Ms. Lewis, I thought, *if I ever get the chance to teach, I'm going to teach in the same way*.

Ms. Lewis previously worked in hospitals and EDs for most of her career, and she often reminisced about the good ol' days of saving lives in the ED. She took me and three others in my cohort to a large nursing home where we would complete our clinical rotation. We showed up, dressed in those terrible all translucent white uniforms—you know, the one with the zipper in the front, the flared-out collar, and the terrible pleats on the back of the shirt. The uniform was awful and a far cry from anything remotely masculine.

Ms. Lewis gave us our assignments. Some people had more than one person to care for, but I had only one for my entire rotation: Darrell. He was a charming Southern man in his 40s, a Jehovah's Witness, neat, organized, very precise about everything, and he knew every detail about his care. Darrell was a quadriplegic, as a result of a gunshot to the head.

Before I met Darrell, my instructor explained many of the things I would need to do to care for him. I'd need to check his blood pressure, set up his food tray, help him get dressed, help him get into his wheelchair, and do pretty much whatever else he needed help with for that day.

Ms. Lewis told me he used a Texas catheter, and showed me how to apply it. To which I replied, "How am I supposed to put that on a man?" Honestly, as a heterosexual man, I was mortified by the idea of putting a condom on another man. She told me, "Darrell will teach you," and he did. He explained why he was incontinent and how the Texas Catheter helped him to be more functional.

Several days a week, for 3 or 4 weeks, I took care of Darrell. I took care of his meals. I checked his vitals. I dressed him in three-piece suits several times a week, so he could attend the kingdom hall. I learned that it was really difficult to dress a 200-pound quadriplegic man in a suit, but it was worth it to him every time. He taught me how to do everything to take care of him—to assist in some basic range of motion exercises to help relieve his muscle spasms, to bathe him and shave his face, to use the lift to load him into his chair for activities, and to take him out of the chair when he was done for the day and put him back in bed. I didn't see much of my instructor during my rotation. She knew Darrell would teach me just about everything I needed to know, and he did. By the end of my rotation Darrell and I had grown pretty close. On the last day of my rotation, Darrell told me that over the past 10 years, he hadn't had anyone care for him the way I did. He told me that I was good at this kind of work and that I should not underestimate the importance of this work.

Whatever difficulty I endured in my duties paled in comparison to the impact I could have on the individual. Whatever effort it took to care for others was truly small compared to the fullness I felt in my heart, knowing I spent my time making a difference.

I spent the next 20 years of my career climbing the professional ladder. I became an LPN, through the most difficult training I've ever completed. I later went on to get my associate degree (RN) and then my bachelor's degree (BSN). I completed my master's degree and training as a nurse practitioner, and eventually completed my training as a nurse scientist (PhD). Along the way, I worked in every kind of setting that would hire me. I worked as a traveling nurse, in ICUs, EDs, medical–surgical units, substance use treatment programs, home health services, and behavioral health. I taught CNA, LPN, RN, and DNP students.

I've been caring for people, patients, colleagues, and students, with the same intention for the past 20 years. I've never forgotten how amazing it feels to empower someone else. Throughout my career, I've had the privilege of seeing our healthcare through the lens of multiple nursing practice levels and various settings. Regardless of what level I practiced, or what setting I was working in, the nurse seemed to have the least amount of power or influence to effectively make positive change. I was frustrated by this, as many nurses are, and wasn't able to escape this feeling of powerlessness.

In recent years, I've found myself working as an organizer to support grassroots nursing movements, such as Show Me Your Stethoscope and Nurses Take DC. These movements are led by bedside nurses advocating for themselves and for the nursing profession. I began writing and speaking about the need to empower nurses as individuals and as professionals at large. An empowered nursing profession is the key to revolutionizing healthcare. This idea ultimately has become my purpose, my life's work, and is my way of giving back to a profession that has given me so much.

My career in healthcare started without an understanding of my purpose and passion. About 20 years later, when people ask why I became a nurse, I tell them that I started my career in healthcare because I was hungry; but I became a NURSE because I strive to be the change I want to see in the world. I tell them my purpose is to be in the service of others and my passion is to create positive change through empowerment and any means necessary.

Here are a few lessons I've learned along my journey.

- A little bit of luck and good connections may bring good fortune. However, honest, diligent work and putting forth 100% effort will eventually bring success. Never underestimate the value of hard work.

- As nurses, our training helps us care for individuals and populations. We are trained to make an impact. Never underestimate the impact you have and always strive to find ways to make your impact broader, deeper, and more meaningful.

- Be brave and ambitious in your assertions. Aim high, for if and when you fail, you will fail forward. A goal not met brings much value and many lessons that will ultimately guide you on your road to success.

A Spark of Inspiration

RHONDA MANNS, MBA, BSN, RN

"OTHERS OFTEN SEE THE GEMS HIDDEN INSIDE OF YOU. DON'T BE AFRAID TO EXPLORE THOSE OPPORTUNITIES. THEY MAY LEAD TO SOME UNEXPECTED DISCOVERIES."

—RHONDA MANNS

It's a miracle that I'm a nurse. It's also a miracle that I can say that I've completed college at the undergraduate and graduate level. My journey into nursing isn't traditional or cliché. I wasn't born into a family of nurses; I don't have a momentous story about encountering a nurse who inspired me through a personal hospitalization or illness. Many of the student nurses and nurse professionals that I mentor know that I never intended to become a nurse. It happened. I mean, it found me. Or I found it; actually, like a romance story, we found each other unexpectedly, at a critical time in my life.

I'll preface this section to say that I'm so glad that life has unfolded in this way. Life is sort of like a tapestry viewed from the backside—all I can see is a scrambled mess of strings, but to the artist, it is a masterpiece.

Born and raised in New York City, my childhood was filled with memories—open fire hydrants in the summer, riding bicycles until the streetlamps turned on, and chasing lightning bugs until midnight. Life was good, fun, carefree—as it should be—until shortly before eighth grade, when everything changed quickly and for the worse. My father was a New York State (NY) police officer. Because of various threats, our family of four was forced to relocate into a two-bedroom apartment with four other family members for our safety and refuge. Abruptly required to transition, we relocated every 2 years. Future planning and longevity were replaced with a constant sense of fight, flight, and survival to meet our most immediate and basic needs.

While I was smart *and athletic*, I listened to my other peers speak about their next steps and graduated high school without a plan of my own for college. I never thought I was smart enough to go to college; so I never considered it, and it certainly didn't cross my mind that I should go. I needed someone to tell me that college was the next step into adulthood, but I never heard such a message. I was the oldest daughter of two professionally employed parents who didn't attend college. Although they sincerely believed in education, career preparation, and certifications, I find it strange that we never planned for anything.

Many years went by, and in that time, I'd tried to become an x-ray technician through a hospital program and failed out in the first semester. I later became an emergency medical technician (EMT) and served at the September 11—World Trade Center site. I then left New York City for New Jersey and joined a hospital trauma team as an ED technician. I wanted to balance my work hours of responding to motor vehicle accidents, heart attacks, and transporting tiny neonatal babies. I became a massage therapist and filled my days with soft music, Tibetan wind chimes, and aromatherapy products. It wasn't until many years later that I was exposed to college and campus life. I visited my younger sister in her on-campus dorm room. The following week I called her and asked what "going to college was like." It was then that I broke down and cried and asked her if she thought that I could do it, too.

I relocated from New Jersey to South Carolina, where I would self-fund my education. I dreamt of becoming a doctor but quickly ran out of money after the first semester. I worked for another 6 months and then transferred from the university's pre-med program into the local community college to continue my studies, when all the stars lined up. Yes, it was kismet.

On the morning that I was due to meet the enrollment advisor, I stepped into the grand lobby of the community college and felt a slight buzz from my phone. I noticed that I had a text message and a separate voice mail that begged for my attention. But that would have to wait, because I was on a mission. I was meeting the admissions counselor to review my transcripts, so that I could take the courses that I needed to transfer back to the university because I had a plan.

I entered the advisor's office and slid my papers across the cherry wood desk. She asked me about my goals and reviewed the forms. Alternating her glances between the forms in her hand and peering over the upper rim of her glasses, she interrupted the moment of awkward silence with a single statement.

"Are you sure you want to be a doctor, because I think you'd be great for the nursing program."

I grinned politely and remained silent until I could figure out how to soften my immediate response.

Internally, I continued the dialogue to myself.

"Nursing? Nursing? I didn't come in here to talk about a nursing program."

I shifted in my seat and continued to myself.

"I've never even considered nursing—even though I've worked with some amazing nurses in Morristown—and yeah, they got to do some really cool stuff, but … no."

"Nursing? No."

"Me? A nurse?"

I grinned again and began to speak when she was called out of the room. I reached into my purse, grabbed my phone, and listened to the voice mail. The deep rich tones of my father's voice blared through the phone's speaker, "Rhonda, I'm worried about you. Listen, I know you're meeting with those school people. Have you thought about becoming a nurse? You know your cousin works at an insurance company and she likes it. Call me back."

A single, unread text message remained. It was from my best friend and former NYC EMT ride-along partner who followed her Naval husband to Virginia. It said, "[something something-something] why don't you just become a nurse?"

I was startled as the admissions counselor reentered the room. Apologizing for the brief break, she said, "So, about nursing … " The synchronicity of these events was perfectly orchestrated.

"Tell me more … " I said with a half-formed smile and semi-whimsical, drawn-out tone.

I needed three more sciences to satisfy the prerequisites for the nursing program. The admissions counselor placed my schedule in a large envelope and told me to complete the nursing application at the end of the semester. Aside from the standard transcript request and demographics form, I was surprised to find out that the application process also included a selective ranking score sheet that assigned point values to each of the grades achieved for the required prerequisite courses. With A's ranking higher than C's for each of the courses, the cumulative point-based system also worked in my favor when I received additional points for having worked as an EMT. And with that, I was accepted into the associate degree of nursing program at Spartanburg Community College.

I graduated at the top of my class with two nursing awards: The peer-based Florence Nightingale Award—given to the student who displayed compassion, commitment to patient care, excellence in nursing studies, and served as an example for others; and the Nurse Leadership Award—presented by the Chief Nursing Officer (CNO) of Mary Black Hospital to a student who demonstrated leadership skills, helpfulness to other students, a positive attitude, responsibility, and resiliency. That night, the CNO offered to meet with me for career exploration and interviews, during a time when there were few nursing positions.

Much of the credit for the beginning of my nursing career came from others who recognized something within me and said, "Go there next." At every pivotal point in my life and my career, I see where someone came forward at just the right time to shine a light on the next step of my pathway. The English teacher who encouraged me to write more stories; the nursing instructor who told me about the Mary Black Foundation scholarship; the college professor who shared her life's wisdom with me; and the assistant nurse manager who recognized my skills, which benefit the department through committees, projects, and other initiatives. I look at the value added by these people, and I see clearly the reasons behind my ongoing commitment to providing career guidance and mentoring to adolescents and young adults.

In my 10 years of nursing tenure, I rose from a new nurse to a charge nurse, preceptor to nurse management. I worked in a variety of settings, from acute inpatient rehab to the ED, and then to pharmaceuticals for rare disease populations and patient education. I've worked as an intravenous (IV) infusion nurse, consultant, and now a case manager—each role teaching me a little bit more about myself, disease processes, nursing science, and the fragility of the human condition. And through each experience, I've rediscovered a new love for different aspects of nursing. My most favorite nurse role was one that gave me a sense of autonomy and combined my clinical knowledge with transitional care management and business communications.

My role as an IV infusion nurse actually led to understanding many of the world's rarest blood, nerve, and immunologic disease states and treatments. And it was in that role where I was able to shift gears to support the account management team in the care delivery for pulmonary hypertension (PH) patients—a rare, progressive cardiopulmonary condition in which the lung's arteries become narrowed, stiff, or occluded, leading to right-sided heart failure and shortness of breath. And while the prognosis may be poor, the PH patient population, caregivers support, and medical community was so closely knitted and unlike anything that I have ever seen or experienced before.

What I learned was that the condition did not discriminate based on money, titles, social standing, age, race, or location. Young, old, Black, White, Asian, Indian, Latinx, children, mothers, wives, sons, husbands, newborns, executives, farm workers, teenagers, and nurses. No one was immune. I've initiated and supported the treatment of patients as young as 2 years old up to a newly diagnosed 93-year-old woman. Day after day, week after week; some weeks driving *at least* 1,000 miles to see patients and assess their well-being and tolerance to medications that supported their condition but could not cure it. And yet, most of these PH patients lived with a sense of gratitude and appreciation that could not be shaken; even on the tough days. It was *in that role* that I realized the power of a nurse who can effectively make a difference in nontraditional patient care delivery environments and corporations. It was then that the limitations of what a nurse can do dissolved right before my eyes. This is why I stand by my life's purpose to find a position that allows me to leverage my clinical knowledge with business acumen to enhance healthcare delivery for positive patient outcomes.

In my career, I have completed a bachelor of science in nursing, summa cum laude, and a graduate master's (MBA) degree with a 4.0 distinction. I stand amazed, because I have the opportunity to create and develop new initiatives in healthcare delivery, or to teach and train others to do their best work. There are moments when you may find me in a room—off to the side, smiling to myself—lost in the thought of where the field of nursing has taken this New York City girl, who didn't think she could accomplish very much at all.

And I smile, because all it took was a spark of inspiration.

- In your career, there will be others who can see the gems hidden inside you; don't be afraid to explore those opportunities, because they may lead to some unexpected discoveries.

- Exposure is the key, so be courageous! Visit new places, speak to new people, and always remain a continual learner. You may fall in love with another element of your role, job, or department, and the next leg of your journey.

- Find a mentor and develop new social circles that can help you appreciate and understand how your life's story adds to your life's purpose.

Be uniquely you. That is *your* superpower.

SUPPLEMENTAL RESOURCES

- Nursing program at Spartanburg Community College
  https://www.sccsc.edu/nursing
- Mary Black Foundation
  https://maryblackfoundation.org
- The Nurses Collective: (Description: mentorship/career advice and social circle for nurses)
  https://www.linkedin.com/groups/8700466
- McBride, A. B. (2020). *The growth and development of nurse leaders* (2nd Ed.). New York, NY: Springer Publishing Company.

Be Exceptional

NICOLE LINCOLN, MS, RN, FNP-BC, CCNS, CCRN

"TO ME THERE IS NO OTHER CAREER ON THE PLANET LIKE NURSING."

As a young child, my mother and father had a traumatic divorce and sadly lost the ability to focus on being parents. My mother abandoned us when I was around 10 years old. She could not cope with the overwhelming pressures of single parenting. My father took over as the custodial parent at that point. This continued in a semistable fashion for the next 2 to 3 years and then tragedy struck again. The two people who had been our rock, my paternal grandparents, died within 6 months, one after the other. After that, it was each man, woman, and child for themselves.

I moved out on my own with friends when I was 16 years old. By the 11th grade, I was a high school dropout. I luckily possessed a very strong work ethic, as I enjoyed working. So quitting school seemed the right route at the time. I worked various jobs during this period, including childcare and fashion retail. One day I took the advice of a friend and began working at a local nursing home. This changed my life forever. I had always loved elderly people. I found peace and reward in taking care of them and spreading laughter. I missed my grandparents so much and this was a way for me to feel connected to them. I had found my purpose in life. I wanted to be a nurse!

I reached back out to my mother after many years of distance. She was a professor at a local community college. She set me up to take my General Education Development (GED) examination and enroll for nursing prerequisites. After successful GED completion, I began going to classes and excelling at the coursework. After a year, my GPA and SAT scores were able to secure me placement in a baccalaureate nursing program. I also met who I thought was the man of my dreams, and fell in love for the first time.

My first semester while living in the dormitory at the new university, I learned I was pregnant with my son. I completed the semester and moved home to give birth at the age of 19. I had a beautiful and healthy son on March 4, 1992. I transferred my nursing credits back home, and was accepted to the nursing program at a local university in Boston. Before I knew it, I was pregnant once again with my daughter, born February 11, 1993. During this period I continued full-time course work in nursing.

Over this time period, things started to deteriorate with "Mr. Right." Once domestic violence began in our home, I decided to go to a homeless shelter for women and children called Wellsprings in Gloucester, Massachusetts. My mother bought me an old beat up Toyota Corolla, and I commuted each day from Gloucester to Boston for classes.

I got subsidized housing from the Section 8 program that gave me stability and an apartment closer to town. This was when I had a real stroke of luck! Through Catholic Charities, I met Claudette, who would be my guardian angel and childcare provider throughout the remainder of my undergraduate studies. She took my infant children at 4:30 a.m. every day, so I could make it to clinical on time. If my car broke down, she would instruct her husband, Al, to come pick us up at 4:00 a.m., so I could go to school. She believed in me. She was my mentor, friend, and mother all wrapped up in one amazing person.

The time came for me to graduate in 1995 with my BSN. Against all odds I had finished; I was a nurse! My kids, dad, mom, and Claudette were all there with me at graduation. My grandmother was there too, as my dad provided me with a corsage to remind me how proud they would be of me on that day. When I was pinned, I pinned Claudette with a golden guardian angel. I was ready for the good life!

I moved to Boston and took my first nursing job at the Lemuel Shattuck Hospital (LSH). The LSH was owned and operated by the State of Massachusetts and focused on public health concerns. A large proportion of the patients at LSH were state prisoners. It was 1995 in the height of the AIDS epidemic. Many of the prisoners were dying from complications of AIDS. This was a crucial point for me as a nurse and a human being. I realized that health alone was something to be grateful for. I became passionate about health equity, death with dignity, and giving the best care I could to those dying inmates.

Three years later in 1998, I took a position in critical care in an ICU at Boston Medical Center (BMC). Almost 21 years later, I continue to work at BMC. It is a place I can call home. The wonderful people I have worked with over the years are like family. The patients and families I have had the pleasure to take care of have meant the world to me. The mission, vision, and values of BMC are aligned with my own personal values. I was able to effectively balance my home life as a single mother and my professional life as a highly skilled ICU nurse. To me there is no other career like nursing on the planet.

In 2011, I decided I was ready for an added layer in my career. I wanted to be a part of innovating the evolution of the nursing profession. In the recent wave of technology, the advancements were monumental. Change was the only thing you could count on in medical care. Some of the changes were not well thought out, and had unintended consequences. There was and is ample room for new workflows, ideas, and innovation. Nurses needed a voice in this movement. They needed a place at the table. I was working as a resource nurse at the time, and wanted to be able to find solutions to the problems nurses were facing every shift while caring for their patients.

I attended graduate school and trained as a critical care clinical nurse specialist (CCNS). This role is focused on the three domains of the American Association of Critical-Care Nurses (AACN) Synergy Model (patient, nurse, system). The CCNS will impact the system at all three levels as a change agent. I graduated with my CCNS in 2014. I then went on to complete a post-masters certification as a family nurse practitioner (FNP). The two roles combined gave me a well-rounded view of quality improvement and as a clinician. It is important to stay relevant in the field to stay close to the patient.

My graduate education was the catalyst for my innovation journey at BMC. I took a full-time position as a nurse educator at BMC. I covered the cardiac and renal inpatient units. I began to focus on safety events that were occurring on my units. The majority of these were related to medication, other medical errors, and falls with injury. The nurse educators at BMC had traditionally focused on the onboarding of new hires. In addition they taught the skills and competencies necessary to adequately perform on the job. My goal was to flip the classroom! I wanted to find out what the nurses thought would be the best solutions to address the quality and safety problems on the units.

The journey started with fall prevention innovation. The frontline nurses had the opportunity to partner with healthcare engineering students and quality improvement specialists to innovate solutions to falls occurring on their units. The nurses came up with the idea to turn the large 36 bed unit into three smaller pods. The assignments were then made geographically within the pod. This innovation reduced the falls on the unit by 76% during the pilot period. The team was excited but resumed traditional nongeographically based care after the 3-month pilot. There was an immediate decline in the falls rate. The frontline nurses huddled and made the decision to shift to pod nursing for the long run. The team won the

Be Exceptional Award. Pod nursing was spread to other units. Nursing innovation at BMC was on its way!

Next came a series of dangerous medication errors on the cardiac unit. Frontline nurses explored evidence-based practice related to medication errors, and determined nursing bedside handoff would provide the solution to their serious problem. They implemented nursing bedside handoff on the unit, and saw a 25% reduction in medication error during the pilot period. They also saw patient experience scores improve dramatically. The entire hospital adopted nursing bedside handoff over the next 2-year period. Patient experience had the highest 6-month scores in history after the adoption of bedside handoff organization-wide.

A whole new universe had opened up for me. Continuing my education had broadened my perspective and given me a new purpose in my career. This taught me to accept that risks are good when you are innovating. As a nurse, my whole career of taking risks was viewed negatively. In innovation, failure is a chance to learn, but in nursing, failure meant possible harm to a patient. I suddenly realized that to reinvent myself, I had to be open to all possibilities.

All of this innovation won the attention of new senior nursing leaders at BMC. This led to the development of a dedicated position to develop and encourage nursing innovation. Frontline nurses are optimally positioned to impact care at the bedside. They are closest to it, and the constant for the patient. Nursing councils were being created at the hospital-wide, as well as unit-based level, to support this work. Nurses were positioned as key players at quality improvement committees. The kickoff for this new focus on nursing innovation took shape as a "Nurse Tank" contest. Nurse Tank was based on the popular show Shark Tank. Nurses at BMC were asked to pitch their patient care improvement ideas. Over 60 nurses, or groups of nurses, came forward with proposals. The proposals went before the Be Exceptional Board of Trustees, including the hospital CEO.

The Nurse Tank event was well received. Board members were thrilled with the ideas nurses presented. Ten projects were ultimately chosen for funding. This was an exciting day for all involved. The success of Nurse Tank led to nurses entering other calls for local improvement and safety grants. Nurses for the first time were the recipients of internal safety grants that had traditionally gone to physician colleagues. Nurses were on the improvement map at BMC and, frankly, beginning to dominate.

This led physician leaders to involve nurses at the leadership level in quality and safety steering committees. I was included in key meetings where a place could be carved out for frontline nurses at each and every initiative. They truly were keys to the success of virtually every effort to improve patient care. Work groups formed of residents and frontline nurses to improve interdisciplinary communication. Doctors and Nurses Communicating Effectively (DANCE) was developed as an interdisciplinary simulations lab scenario. Work to improve rounding on all of the units was underway.

Collaboration of the interdisciplinary team is key to the success of an organization. Shared governance is also important to create a just culture where people are not afraid to speak up. Most recently, nurses are working with physicians, physical therapy/occupational therapy (PT/OT), pharmacy, and all other key stakeholders to redesign the way care is given. The interdisciplinary team has created an Improvement Leadership Academy (ILA) for learners to have support and formal quality improvement training during the implementation of their project ideas. Graduates have presented at national conferences. Nurses and physicians at BMC collaborated to publish a patient safety book "OK to Proceed?" There have been major strides in the reduction of the preventable harm index and mortality observed-to-expected ratio. This can only be done when all members of a team feel they have a significant voice.

Currently nurses, medical students, and residents are partnering to plan upcoming hackathon events. These events will lead to the development of a fresh batch of innovations. As we move forward, a next step will be to add nursing innovation, business, and entrepreneurship education to new graduate residency programs at BMC. Nurses must be empowered to shape care at the bedside. They are leaving the bedside at alarming rates. Healthcare is fragmented, and nurses as the end users feel the brunt of this—more than anyone else besides the patient. Asking nurses for solutions to these problems is key to the survival of the profession and our patients!

Another passion I have is in helping women facing economic or societal struggles reach their professional and personal goals. The nursing profession has changed the trajectory of my life forever. Nursing has bestowed gifts upon me that I can never pay back; they are called independence, joy, pride, self-esteem, and purpose. I believe paving the way for women of diverse backgrounds will be key to saving the role of the bedside nurse. Life struggles when overcome are often accompanied with the development of strength, problem-solving ability, creativity, and resiliency. Resilient nurses are needed to manage the demands of bedside nursing and to come up with the solutions needed to reshape care. It is my hope that we will prioritize the recruitment of underserved and minority women into the nursing profession.

SONSIEL has been an exciting venture this far. I am grateful to share in the joy and the possibilities this society will surely offer many nurses in the years to come. The level of interest from entrepreneurs in nursing ideas and innovation is refreshing. These partnerships open up endless possibilities. Nurses will be key stakeholders in health policy and the total redesign of our healthcare delivery model. Nurses must firmly believe in themselves. There were people in my humble beginnings that believed in me. I surely would not be here today if that wasn't the case. All nurses must receive the training needed to compete in the business of healthcare and the tools they need to succeed. It is our job as leaders to open the doors for them, to cultivate these opportunities at all levels both locally and globally. When nurses speak up, the world will surely listen.

SUPPLEMENTAL RESOURCES

- Lemuel Shattuck Hospital

  https://www.mass.gov/locations/lemuel-shattuck-hospital

- Boston Medical Center

  https://www.bmc.org

- BMC: Improvement Leadership Academy

  https://primarycare.hms.harvard.edu/primary-care-improvement-network

- *OK TO PROCEED?*

  https://oktoproceed.com

- Myers, S. A. (2012). *Patient safety and hospital accreditation: A model for ensuring success.* New York, NY: Springer Publishing Company.

- McAllister, M., & Lowe, J. (2011). *The Resilient Nurse: Empowering Your Practice.* New York, NY: Springer Publishing Company.

- Duffy, M., Dresser, S., & Fulton, J. S. (2016). *Clinical Nurse Specialist toolkit: A guide for the new Clinical Nurse Specialist.* (2nd ed.). New York, NY: Springer Publishing Company.

- AACN Synergy Model

  https://www.aacn.org/nursing-excellence/aacn-standards/synergy-model

- Leik, M. T. C. (2018). *Family nurse practitioner certification intensive review: Fast facts and practice questions.* (3rd ed.). New York, NY: Springer Publishing Company.
- Wittmann-Price, R. A., Godshall, M., Wilson, L. (2019). *Certified Nurse Educator (CNE) review manual.* (3rd ed.). New York, NY: Springer Publishing Company.

Nursoldier

SHAILADI GUPTA, BSCN, RN

"LIFE BECOMES A LEGACY WHEN IT IS LIVED FOR A PURPOSE."

I am a mother of a toddler and an infant, a boy and a girl. I have a loving and supporting husband, and I currently reside happily in the heavenly country of Canada. However, I grew up in India, and I never thought that real people are kind and transparent. Fortunately for me, at the core of my nursing profession, my life unfolded into a journey with invaluable relationships. These relationships: with my parents, family, teachers, nursing professors, mentors, patients, colleagues, employers, and many more who crossed the pathway in my life till now, have shaped and refined my character as a woman. They brought greater effectiveness, reputation, and loyalty. One such personality was Dr. Nancy Hanrahan, who was previously leading the innovation and technology development program at the University of Pennsylvania School of Nursing. God serendiptiously connected me with Dr. Nancy Hanrahan, as well as Rebecca Love and Noah Hendler, nurse innovators and entrepreneurs and founders of SONSIEL, in March 2019, and I ended up attending SONSIEL's The Healthcare Innovation Conference (THINC) in Boston, in the United States. THINC was a platform to connect with unique individuals.

However, to understand the uniqueness of where I am, it's important to understand the life I came from. As Swami Vivekanand says, "*You have to grow from the inside out. None can teach you, none can make you spiritual. There is no other teacher but your own soul.*" Life has a black pitch sense of humor. Just when we think life is getting stable, life unveils something, making us realize how little control we have on our lives. This defines my whole life with a major part of it revolving around India, my home land, where my heart belongs.

Since I opened my eyes in this world, I always found myself surrounded by patients, as both of my parents were doctors. I was all too familiar with the healthcare field and glimpses of those who were sick and in need. However, getting into nursing wasn't even my farthest of dreams. I studied in one of the top-notch schools and was trained by the best. I was full of competitive spirit and was a high functioning student, along with prize-winning skills in public speaking, swimming, singing, and dancing.

In regards to the nursing status in India, no one thinks of going into nursing by choice, especially if you are born in a family full of physicians. Although, there are many career options available to nurses. I used to regret this profession in my early years of nursing, I see now that preparation and destiny were at work. The lack of a mentoring culture, and the brutal treatment by some of the professors, left me drained and depressed. During my second year of nursing school, my mother received a diagnosis of colon cancer, turning my life upside down. My mother, a gynecologist, was treated by her nurses like she had committed some sinful act and got cancer because of *karma*. One of the nurses told my mother when she was experiencing the many side effects of chemotherapy to stop acting out and get her IV done quickly. This close exposure to the realities of nursing in India left my mind permanently scarred.

In the same year, I packed my bags and decided to leave the nursing profession. My father took some time out and sat with me to find my vision and a career path. Were it not for my father, I would have lost this opportunity to be a part of such a wonderful, nurturing profession. My professor, Ms. Avinash Rana, often told me to reiterate "I am a nurse" in front of a mirror 10 times a day to make myself believe that I can do it.

In my third year of nursing school, I was posted in community health nursing, which is not what it should be in India. There is no emphasis on patient-centered care. One of the families I was attending to included eight family members, all living in a single room, cooking, and smoking, even with children and a pregnant woman. There were cases of domestic abuse that were not resolved, and there was nothing we could do about it. There were no suggestions we could give for advanced or specific care. As a nurse, I felt helpless and pointless, unable to offer any real help with my visits. Working in the labor and delivery room revealed more bitter truths. Multiple expecting mothers would be placed in a single room with no drapes or privacy, left to be seen by each other's family members.

In my final year of nursing school, my mom had another relapse of cancer. This time, it hit us like a tsunami, leaving us all dismantled. She underwent surgery again, and was left with a colostomy bag, but there was no health education related to colostomy care. Cancer is considered a terminal condition, and nursing care is focused on the coping of the patient and family members. But, no nurse thought of asking my father how he was managing the weight on his shoulders. The oncologist recommended radiation therapy for the growing tumor, while some sort of medical negligence led to her getting adhesions in her intestines, increasing her pain and trauma. My father made every effort to give us a normal life, but I knew this trauma was never going to end.

I migrated to Canada for my higher studies in 2009, where I came across a different continuum of the nursing profession, one with more focus on a holistic approach, therapeutic communication, and patient- and family-centered care. Along with my personal growth, I learned to accept and appreciate the support of my fellow nurses throughout my entire process of developing transformative competencies of leadership. I was hired as an RN in Extendicare Long-Term Care home in Toronto soon after I got my license, with my second job being in a Slimband bariatric surgery clinic. My quest for knowledge was not being fulfilled as I sifted through jobs; however, I gained enough experience while working at long-term care homes to transition through different roles and positions. I loved working at the bedside, and my patients still remember my name as someone who actually cared and courageously solved their problems. But I always felt like I was missing something. It was like my intuition was telling me that I was needed somewhere else.

My next adventure was working at Seneca College of Applied Arts and Technology, where I joined as a professor for coronary care nursing and worked as a coordinator for the nursing leadership and management program for international nursing students. I was personally well-versed with struggles of internationally educated nurses (IEN) in a new country, but it was after working in a close relationship with these nurses that I was led to understand how much they actually needed assistance from someone who has lived the same journey. This gave me strength to start Kindshell, a project specifically designed for IENs to help them through the complicated process of becoming a nurse in Canada and the United States. Kindshell has worked toward helping IENs through the steps of licensing, along with entering the nursing profession equipped with the right tools, keeping in mind the job burnout they may face while working.

My vision is to provide nurses around the world with the tools and education to make a difference every day. I envision a newfound respect for the nursing profession in my incredible homeland of India, so that no nurse leaves the country. Although my life journey has had the trajectory of an ordinary human being with the same opportunities as every other nurse in India, my ongoing hope and tenacity have led me to something wonderful. Life becomes a legacy when it is lived for a purpose.

SUPPLEMENTAL RESOURCES

- THINC Conference

  https://www.facebook.com/events/umass-boston/thinc-the-healthcare-innovation-conference/349663775635376

- University of Pennsylvania School of Nursing

  https://www.nursing.upenn.edu

- Rosa, W. (2017). *A new era in global health: Nursing and the United Nations 2030 Agenda for Sustainable Development.* New York, NY: Springer Publishing Company.

- Curley, A. L. *Population-based nursing: Concepts and competencies for advanced practice.* (3rd Ed.). New York, NY: Springer Publishing Company.

  https://www.springerpub.com/population-based-nursing-second-edition-9780826196132.html

---

The Nursing Opportunity

BONGI SIBANDA, DNPc, MSc, ANP, FHEA, RN

"I AM CONSTANTLY REMINDED OF THE REASON I ENTERED THE NURSING PROFESSION—TO SERVE AND MAKE A DIFFERENCE WITH EXCELLENCE."

"I am pleased to inform you that you have been selected to be one of the American Association of Nurse Practitioners (AANP) International Ambassadors ... " read a line on an email in early 2018, a line that was not only a professional triumph, but also one that had profound meaning to my personal life and, to date, the most extraordinary award. Without a shadow of doubt, I knew this couldn't be luck; but rather, it was the result of hard work and opportunities graced upon me in life. I would utilize this opportunity to the best of my ability and help serve a wider community, including the African continent. We have seen significant progress toward the development of APRN and midwifery roles in Africa as part of our Anglophone Africa APRN Coalition: a community of global experts working with international organizations, African nurse leaders, policymakers, healthcare practitioners, academics, colleagues, and African communities across relevant disciplines to help advance the APRN/midwife agenda in Africa. This is an "American dream" in a true sense, despite the fact that I live mainly in the United Kingdom and Zimbabwe. Let me take you back to the 1990s to help you understand this extraordinary leadership journey from a Zimbabwean–British nurse who has seen every struggle, defied what statistics say about those from single-parent homes or who are orphaned, and continues to overcome challenges in pursuit of excellence in nursing and education.

I had been labeled as exceptionally gifted in childhood, and my mom (a former teacher) had secured an American scholarship for me, or so she thought. After months of a rigorous selection process, mom went to collect final papers for the approved scholarship, only to find that my name had been removed and replaced with another child's from a different region in the country. That evening, mom came home with tears in her eyes. As she relayed her day trip to her eldest daughter, tears continued to run down. The injustice, betrayal, and hard work of a single mom in preparation for this American scholarship washed away. At that moment, as a head girl in my primary school at the time, I helped her to see the way forward, to continue to believe in me, and to remember that God has His timing—this time it was not mine.

This setback did not mean much to me. I was enjoying my time at school, consistently helping my teacher in class and supporting my peers when I finished my own work ahead of schedule. What mattered most to me over the years had not been the number of accolades I collected each term in primary school; but rather, seeing my peers improve their marks, class positions, or their performances in drama. This setback was a blessing in disguise that allowed me to do what I love throughout my years. Ultimately, I became a nurse after high school, fulfilling my childhood ambition.

Unfortunately, mom did not live to see me become a nurse; at the age of 37, she left this world. A teenager at the time and the oldest sibling in a single-parent home, I became the leader of the home with the responsibility of caring for my younger siblings. To date, this has been the most challenging responsibility I have had. I made many personal and professional sacrifices along the way to look after my siblings, but these choices overwhelmingly shaped my nursing leadership journey. At the age of 37, I was awarded the AANP scholarship award. Looking back, had I been successful in moving to the United States through the scholarship my mom had pursued, I could have pursued a different career and missed the opportunity to appreciate life as it is seen through the lens of nursing.

Since qualifying as registered general nurse (RGN) at age 20 in Zimbabwe, I have held a number of roles, including working in a pediatric mental health hospital, multiple clinical research projects, intensive care, and emergency care. In the early 2000s, I moved to the United Kingdom to further my career. Following a nurse adaptation, I secured a substantive post in emergency care in Surrey. I fell in love with the specialty—the pace, the diversity of patients, and the proximity to a major airport. However, I wanted to move to a major tertiary hospital where I could have the opportunity to build on my expertise in emergency care. I intentionally started to study at St. George's Hospital (SGH) in Tooting, South West London, a major trauma, cardiac, and stroke center at the time. At times, I would transfer critically ill patients from our ED in Surrey to the resuscitation room at SGH, and each time, I knew I wanted to work there. I visited the St. George's University of London, a campus co-located with the hospital, knowing that I wanted to study there, too. And I did, specializing in emergency care, trauma, and prescribing.

In my third year of working at SGH ED as a senior staff nurse, my matrons and consultant nurse selected me as a junior member of staff to attend an emergency nursing conference in Harrogate with the senior leadership team. The trip changed my career trajectory, and contributed immensely to what I do now as an advanced nurse practitioner in primary and emergency care, and as an educator. The advanced practice education and roles described were exactly what I wanted to do in nursing—to stay in clinical practice while building excellence in research, education, and leadership.

Later that year, I commenced my MSc advanced nurse practitioner (primary care) degree at Queen Mary University of London (QMUL). Although I left SGH ED in 2011, upon qualifying as an advanced nurse practitioner at QMUL, I remain a prodigal daughter to the department, and most colleagues who worked in that department will share the same sentiments. We were a family at work—innovative practice was encouraged through exceptional leadership in our ED. It's important to choose your employer wisely. A good employer will see your potential and offer you opportunities that will help you succeed in your career. Opportunities matter—one can be exceptional, but if that potential is not realized, nothing will ever come to fruition.

I have had the privilege to serve in a number of regional and international nursing roles for the past 6 years, including a membership in the International Council of Nurses Advanced Practice Nursing Network (APNN), as a policy leader for the Africa Interprofessional Education Network (AfrIPEN), and as an NHS Research Ethics Committee expert member. I also held a number of high-level consultancy roles and senior roles in higher education and clinical practice. However, I often faced discrimination, bullying, and jealousy in many of these roles. I have been excluded in meetings discussing my ideas and have been "forced to resign" from jobs I love, because those in authority wanted to take over my projects. While it was difficult during those challenging times, I have learned that these situations arise because of something bigger, more meaningful, and more worthy of my energy around the corner. Whenever we do something extraordinary, something outside the norm, we will face opposition, challenges, and doubt—from ourselves and from others. It is important to be surrounded by those who have a similar energy and aim toward success.

I am truly honored to have found SONSIEL, a family of like-minded nurses pushing boundaries and challenging the status quo to redefine nursing and its meaning. As I build on my work as an AANP International Ambassador and my newly formed social enterprise, APRN Africa CIC (community interest company), to help develop advanced nursing and midwifery practice roles in London and Africa, I am constantly reminded of the reason I entered the nursing profession—to serve and make a difference with excellence. It is my hope that we will always be reminded of this, even during trying times. Let's not be afraid to stand out and make it happen for ourselves and those we serve, because we are all unique individuals with so much to give.

SUPPLEMENTAL RESOURCES

- St George's Hospital (SGH)
  https://www.stgeorges.nhs.uk
- Queen Mary University of London (QMUL)
  https://www.qmul.ac.uk
- International Council of Nurses Advanced Practice Nursing Network (APNN)
  https://international.aanp.org
- Africa Interprofessional Education Network (AfrIPEN)
  https://afripen.org

Wake-Up Giant

ANDREA JARAMILLO, BSN, RN

"NURSES ARE PIVOTAL IN HELPING PEOPLE TRANSITION IN THE MOST VULNERABLE MOMENTS
OF LIFE, AS BRIDGES BETWEEN THE RIGIDITY OF SCIENCE AND THE FLEXIBILITY OF THE ARTS."

This story is dedicated to first generations, to people who embrace change. To the ones who challenge the status quo: the visionaries, the thinkers and troublemakers. The unicorns in the room, the wild spirits. The activists and advocates, the risk takers, the brave. To every nurse who thinks differently and inspires change; to every nurse who is ready to rekindle their fire. You will conquer your fears, persevere, find your voice and rise.

There I was, holding a piece of paper that would mark a before and an after. My hands were shaking. I was feeling every heartbeat pounding in my chest. This piece of paper could make me feel human again. My "green card" (permanent resident card) was that piece of paper, a green light to having an American dream. I was entangled in a broken immigration system—in limbo for several years. My family suddenly needed to migrate to the United States when I was 16. I encountered the bureaucracy of becoming a citizen. My mom, an American by birth, had migrated as a child to Ecuador, where I was born and raised. I was told that I was first in line. Although my case was deemed a priority, as a single child of an American citizen, this process took several years. I used to think of those years as lost, as if I had been left behind.

I can remember the difficulty of navigating systems without a proper identification, without a network, without knowing. Stumbling in the dark. I can remember being the patient without health insurance, the language discordant patient, the one with housing and food insecurity. Still, there I was, determined to become a nurse. Nurses are pivotal in helping people transition in the most vulnerable moments of life, as bridges between the rigidity of science and the flexibility of the arts. They are witnesses of broken systems—systems that play with the human condition. I could identify with nurses; I realized that immigrants and nurses have a lot in common. They can feel invisible, underrepresented, and often powerless. Yet they share common traits: they are undeniably strong, extremely resourceful, and have power by numbers. Nurses are the cornerstone of the entire healthcare system, while immigrants are the backbone of the American society. I saw nurses as advocates, activists, and most importantly as catalysts of change. I could see the giant sleeping without regard to its own power. I could see the giant—ready to wake up.

My nursing journey started at a community college in Albuquerque, New Mexico. My advisor told me that my grades and my English skills were not good enough to apply to nursing school, but I was not going to let that stop me. I made sure I took every English class I could. I practiced every day. I watched lots of movies, read many books, and studied every word. When I turned 18, my mom returned to Ecuador. My older sister was living in Washington, DC, and I moved in with her. I had $300 in my pocket. We rented a one-bedroom apartment.

I began taking classes at another community college in Rockville, Maryland. I needed to prove that my English was good enough to become a nurse. I volunteered at the National Institutes of Health, where I was trained as a bilingual interpreter. There I worked side by side with doctors and nurses and I was inspired by the care that nurses provided. I realized that being of service does not equate to servitude. My language skills could help people access and understand their healthcare options. I became the bridge between patients and systems.

Many patients looked toward biomedical research, because they did not have access to other healthcare options. I realized people were struggling to find care and that their access to healthcare was not seen as a human right. I realized that becoming a nurse was going to be much more than caring and holding hands. The nursing profession was going to give me a platform to work toward equity and to advocate for the most vulnerable.

I met Pablo in 2010. He was a young doctor from Ecuador who was applying to get into a medical residency program. He inspired me—he worked so hard to relearn everything he learned in med-school in another language. He had grit, passion, and a clear mission to make this world a better place. I admired him and fell in love with everything he was. Nothing we did was done alone: he became my team, my mentor, my family. He believed in me and my vision for nurses to have a bigger impact on society. We moved to Detroit, Michigan for his program. I restarted my classes, this time at a 4-year college. We got married. While he was training to be a doctor, I worked as a nursing assistant at night. I also had the opportunity to be part of a team to improve access for Spanish-speaking patients. I entered the quality improvement world, collaborating in the creation of a clinic for people who preferred to receive their care in their own language. Dr. Chueca took me under her wing. We developed and implemented a model in which patients had access to providers and ancillary staff that spoke their preferred language. I became her medical assistant at the Clínica en Español. The clinic operated at the Internal Medicine clinic at Henry Ford Hospital in Detroit, Michigan. In 2014, we presented our work at Henry Ford Hospital Quality Expo, and our project received the Quality Expo Award and Equity Award. Once some of the members of the team relocated to other cities, the clinic was not able to continue its operations. Pablo finished his residency program and it was time for me to apply to nursing school. He found a program in Boston to specialize in preventive medicine. I applied to many programs in the New England area.

I was rejected seven times. Rejection letters continued to flood my mailbox. Every time an envelope arrived, I would hold it very tight to my heart, close my eyes, and imagine the future. I was told it was very unlikely to get a spot in a nursing program as a transfer student. My sense of worth was shaken. But I did not give up. I continued to apply until I was finally accepted into a bachelor's program in Boston. Each letter served as a reminder to keep persevering in the face of rejection or decline. If you stay in the race long enough, you will find a yes at the end of the road. I couldn't believe I was finally going to become a nurse. I was thrilled!

Nursing school became my playground and the perfect space to experiment. I asked candid questions, showed up at meetings where I was not expected—I brought my own chair. I realized that nurses are expected to be obedient, to follow orders and protocols, and not to question authority. There is no room for failure or mistakes. We are not encouraged to challenge the status quo, to speak out loud, or to innovate. We are made to be good test takers. Nevertheless, nursing school was also the place where I met amazing people. My classmates became my friends, my inspiration, and my constant support. They were a refreshing stream of ideas— discussions about healthcare, social justice issues, and new visions of the future of our world.

My first summer, I was very lucky to meet Jean, a professor in the nursing department who gave me a summer job as her research assistant. She believed in me and she showed me how nurses can use research to impact their communities. She taught me the connection between nursing and policy, she gave me a voice, and she became my role model. She helped me understand how social inequalities affect health and showed me how nurses can advocate for the communities they serve. That summer, in collaboration with the Mauricio Gastón Institute, we collected data related to health insurance literacy and access to healthcare in hard-to-reach Hispanic populations. We gave our community a voice. Under the Affordable Care Act, we helped people enroll in health insurance plans, understand their benefits, and gain access to care.

During my second year, I met Adrianna, a PhD student and a member of the Hispanic Nurses Association. I saw myself in her. She inspired me. She invited me to participate in a leadership program she created for millennial Hispanic nurses. She showed us how to create a brand for ourselves, to network, to lean in without fear. She empowered us to share our ideas, sit at the table, and find opportunities to grow professionally. As I courageously leaned in, I was elected class representative for my cohort and advocated in department meetings for the interests of students. I became the interim treasurer for the National Association of Hispanic Nurses—Boston, applied for dozens of scholarships, and participated in the Hausman Nursing fellowship at Massachusetts General Hospital. I armed myself with knowledge, with courage, and with the unbelievable support of the people surrounding me. I was ready to become a nurse.

In 2017, I graduated with honors. I got my first job in a new graduate program as a labor and delivery nurse. My first year as a nurse was challenging and exciting. After my first year, I assessed my career and how I envisioned my future. I could taste the burnout, the unsustainable work environment, and the unclear path for growth. As many new and experienced nurses, I felt disenchanted with nursing. I realized that becoming a nurse was an act of bravery. To choose a profession that has historically been perceived as subordinate—limited by powerlessness and invisibility—takes vision, courage, and determination. I became fascinated with the dynamics of my role as a bedside nurse. My spirit of inquiry started to surface again. I experimented with the power of nurses at the bedside and how we can influence change at different levels. I implemented innovative evidence-based projects. My first project was the use of music for laboring patients. I always thought of music and sound to be a powerful healing tool. I did some research and found evidence for the use of music to support the management of pain and the overall birthing experience. I got several stakeholders engaged, got a donation to buy speakers, and we started using music as part of our nursing interventions and care. I also received a grant at my institution to colead a safety project. I worked with interdisciplinary and interdepartmental teams to expand our current team trainings. I joined the Integrative Nursing Council and Pain task force at my institution, and became a language and culture consultant for research projects, while continuing to advocate for immigrant rights and women's health issues. I could clearly see how bedside nurses could influence change regardless of challenges and perceived lack of influence. We are experts in the science and the art of caring, and when nurses talk, people listen. We are trusted and are powerful by numbers. We have a voice.

At this early stage of my career, I can clearly envision the future of nursing. SONSIEL and the many amazing nurses who are already working to change the world are serving as healthcare influencers and change agents to solve current and future problems. SONSIEL has given me the opportunity to lead the first cohort of fellows and has provided me with the support and mentorship I need to succeed. There are unlimited possibilities to the role of a nurse. We are building what is possible as we fly the plane. Sometimes this might feel uncomfortable, as if we are in the dark. Remember you are not alone: there are approximately 4 million nurses in the United States and many more around the world caring for the health of humans.

We, the nurses, are no longer sleeping. We are conscious of our power and our voice. We are the giant awakening. We are ready to rise.

SUPPLEMENTAL RESOURCES

- Leonard, G. (1992). *Mastery: The keys to success and long-term fulfillment*: New York, NY: Plume.
- Prather, H. (1983). *Notes to myself: My struggle to become a person*. New York, NY: Bantam.
- Frankl, V. E. (2006). *Man's search for meaning* by Viktor E. Frankl. Boston, MA: Beacon.

- English classes at local community colleges

  Central New Mexico Community College https://www.cnm.edu

  Montgomery College https://www.montgomerycollege.edu
- Royal, B. (2004). *The Little Red Writing Book*. Cincinnati, OH: Writer's Digest Book.

  https://www.amazon.com/Little-Red-Writing-Book/dp/1582975213/ref=sr_1_4?keywords =red+book+of+grammar&qid=1565046208&s=books&sr=1-4
- Volunteering at the NIH Clinical Center

  https://cc.nih.gov/volunteers/opportunities.html
- University of Massachusetts Boston Return to Home Page

  https://www.umb.edu
- The Hispanic Nurses Association

  https://www.nahnnet.org
- Boston Medical Center Integrative Nursing Council

  https://www.bmc.org/medical-professionals/nursing/shared-governance/councils/ integrative-nursing-council

The Rebel Nurse's Progress Note

Though these journeys involve extreme difficulties and challenges, each of them highlight the unwavering strength of every individual's unique story and vision. Though life may require bravery and confidence to guide ambitions, one's hope should go on untouched with the reminder of what's at stake. In order to improve the realm of healthcare, the pure intentions of nurses everywhere must overcome adversity and misfortune.

With such strong numbers, nurses are able to collaborate and form positive relationships to help get through the inevitable hard times. By surrounding yourself with those of similar energy and zeal, you can both inspire others and gather the motivation needed to realize your own potential. These partnerships will help guide you, and build your resilience, as you navigate the unexpected twists, turns, and rejections you may encounter. In this way, your strength, and the strength of others, may help pave the way for you to break new ground, as you change the landscape of healthcare, and ultimately the care that you are able to deliver to others.

Where have you overcome seemingly impossible odds? How can this propel your rebel nurse journey forward?

Transforming Your Passion: Innovatively Adaptive Nurses Working Across Multiple Sectors

To transform, to evolve, to shift and think outside the box is like a metamorphosis. There are struggles, there are self-doubts, there may be growing pains, but there is a beautiful transformation of something new, innovative, and with the ability to impact multiple spheres of influence. Disruptors throughout the many segments of healthcare continue to energize their communities, and make dramatic changes throughout all systems. By partnering with multiple sectors, you can modify the environment of proactive care to enhance health and healing. A growing number of nurses are prime candidates for innovative roles, but they require the adequate tools to get started—tools you can find throughout the following stories. These nurses share their inspiring stories of taking the essence of nursing and transforming it into something new, showing the world that nursing is not limited to settings or situations; rather, once a nurse, always a nurse. These nurses are entrepreneurs, inventors, influencers, and game-changers. These are their rebel nurse *stories.*

The Unforeseen Journey

SHEILA DAVIS, DNP, ANP-BC, FAAN

"IT WAS MY FIGHT, JUST AS IT SHOULD HAVE BEEN EVERYONE'S FIGHT."

I did not grow up wanting to be a nurse. I worked as a candy striper for a few months during my freshman year of high school and distinctly remember telling my mother that "I could never be a nurse. What a horrible job." Then one day, during my senior year in high school, I woke up and declared I was applying to the BSN program at the University of Maine in Orono. Everyone, including myself, was shocked. I wish I could say that it was divine intervention, or that after months of deliberation, I had carefully chosen to be a nurse, but that would not be true. I just decided to be a nurse, and that decision was the beginning of an incredible journey.

After a difficult start to my freshman year at the University of Maine, I decided to find a change of scenery to reset my sights on what was important. Although my family did not think a move away from the familiar was the answer, I was determined to find the environment I was longing for. After deferring for a semester because of a lack of on-campus housing, I arrived at Northeastern University in January of 1985 and began classes at the School of Nursing shortly after. Northeastern was the right fit for me, and I did very well academically from that point on. The school is known for its co-op program and the opportunity to work during the program was a big financial help. Most importantly, those with whom I worked, and those I observed throughout my first co-op, molded my evolving views of the world of nursing.

The impactful relationship I had with my assigned nurse, Jim, grew through the many hours we spent together on and off the floor. Jim's partner, Sam, had recently been diagnosed with AIDS. In these early days of the AIDS epidemic, there was a lot of fear regarding transmission, making Sam's experience more complicated than it had to be. As an inpatient at a local Boston hospital, Sam was close enough for Jim and me to visit regularly. The lack of care Sam received from his nursing team was disheartening. The examples of neglect and recurrent lack of compassion from my future colleagues stuck with me, even when I left, and to the point that it made me contemplate leaving nursing.

However, there were some exceptions to this. One of the nurse's aides, originally from Haiti, was loving and caring, singing to Sam in Creole while she bathed him. That image, like so many from that time, also remains burned in my memory. Joyce was a nurse who came into Sam's room every day, where she greeted Sam first, then addressed Jim and me. This was unique and, although he was often confused or had his eyes closed, Joyce continued to treat Sam as a person who deserves dignity and respect. Joyce also recognized Jim as Sam's long-term partner, with all of the respect afforded that role in someone's life. These were the nurses who inspired me to continue working in HIV care.

This transition marked the beginning of a strange, intense, and amazing time in my life. Before moving to Boston, I had never met anyone who was openly gay. Through my relationship with Jim and Sam and my advocacy efforts for better care and treatment for people with HIV infection, I became a part of the gay community. It was a world very different from my own, and there could have easily been suspicion or lack of inclusion, but that didn't happen. I was included in the happy times, celebrations, holidays and the day-to-day of ordinary life. While grieving is typically very personal and individualized within small groups, both formally and informally, I went to funerals, sat shiva and went to more celebrations of life than I could ever count. These experiences were an important aspect of my own personal growth—my ability to cope and grieve. This community welcomed me, just as many other communities would as my career path migrated around the world.

But this path was not an easy one. As an HIV nurse in the late 1980s and early 1990s, my patients and I continually experienced discrimination and were stigmatized by others. People could not understand why a straight, White woman would choose to join a fight that had "nothing to do with me." How wrong those people were. It *was* my fight, just as it should have been everyone's fight. In 1988, I stumbled upon the Association of Nurses in AIDS Care (ANAC), which became a necessary lifeline for me. Within ANAC, I found my mentors, my heroes, my tribe, and my friends. There were no books about how to deliver HIV care. It was evolving in front of us and we taught each other. We learned from our patients, who were cohesively challenging the way patients and the gay community were involved in advocacy and clinical research. The drug approval process was forever changed by the relentless action of the HIV community. The drug approval process had been a very long process that required years, if not a decade or more, for a drug to be available for patients. There were no approved drugs for HIV treatment in the 1980s and early 1990s, and people were dying at an alarming rate with no options for treatment. This was considered an emergency for the HIV community, and there was a coordinated effort using activism to push the Federal Drug Administration (FDA) to address the issue. New processes were developed that allowed for expedited approval of drugs to provide lifesaving treatments.

In 1991, I was holding my 2-month-old beautiful daughter Eva when Magic Johnson announced he was HIV positive. HIV was still considered a "gay" disease and was hidden in the African American community. Many of us in the HIV community held our breath, hoping that HIV would finally emerge from the shadows, bringing outreach into that hard-hit community.

From that day forward, my daughter enlisted into the fight for justice for the vulnerable. Because I was a single mother, Eva grew up as a permanent fixture in the Boston HIV community. She accompanied me to evening and weekend community events, shared meals with the IV drug-using recovery community, and marched in protests and parades. She remains at my side to this day. I am very proud of the young woman she is now and, while sharing her mom with the HIV community was not easy, she responded with grace and compassion.

Rather than making strategic career moves toward a specific position, I followed my gut. I was open to opportunities for growth and holistic education, while consistently pursuing my quest for social justice. During my years as an RN in the HIV community, I worked in an inpatient HIV unit, in a prison unit, in a clinical trials unit as a nurse, and in community organization. Following these experiences, I went back to school to become an adult nurse practitioner (ANP) at Massachusetts General Hospital (MGH) Institute of Health Professions. The pathophysiology and the challenges of diagnostics and complex treatment of HIV infection were consistently evolving, and I wanted to gain additional education and skills to provide more comprehensive care for my patients. I worked as an ANP at the MGH Infectious Diseases Unit from 1997 to 2014, where I bore witness to a miraculous shift in HIV treatment—from palliative and end-of-life care to treating it as a chronic disease. During my years at MGH, I was able to work in parts of Africa where the tragic reality of global health inequity steered me to my next career shift.

In 2010, I joined Partners In Health (PIH), an international nongovernmental organization (NGO) that fights injustice by working to provide healthcare in partnership with local communities throughout 10 countries globally. It was my first position that went beyond HIV—an opportunity to highlight the role of nurses who provide care in low resource settings. In 2014, the Ebola virus was taking hold in West Africa and the global community was not responding to their calls for help. Although not an emergency organization, PIH responded to the moral imperative and committed to going into Sierra Leone and Liberia to fight Ebola. For PIH, it was a challenging time, as we had never responded to an emergency in uncharted territory. The many possible dangers to first responders made the situation even more complicated. These efforts needed a systems leader—someone who could build teams, multitask, and thrive in chaos—so I stepped up and volunteered to lead PIH's response in both countries. The decision by PIH leadership was a complete leap of faith. Although I had successfully implemented PIH nursing programs for the past 4 years, this new effort was unprecedented. Finances and reputations of the staff and the entire organization were at risk.

The PIH team worked successfully in both Sierra Leone and Liberia in collaboration with local governments and other NGO partners to combat Ebola. At the very beginning, we committed to staying long-term in both countries to help rebuild health systems after the end of the outbreak. Ebola was a symptom of a broken health system—to leave without fighting to provide a new primary health system and a safe place for mothers to give birth was out of the question. We have remained in both countries to this day. My role in leading PIH's Ebola response led to other leadership opportunities within PIH, and in June of 2019, I was named PIH's CEO. A nurse CEO of a Harvard-affiliated, physician-centric, 17,000-person NGO was as much of a surprise to me as it was to the rest of the global health community. A dear colleague of mine from Rwanda told me that his daughter overheard him talking about the CEO announcement when she asked what a CEO was. He was so happy that his daughter's first image of a CEO was not only a woman, but a nurse.

As with my decision to become a nurse, I wish I was able to say that I was driven to step up and lead PIH's Ebola response because of divine intervention or after a careful and in-depth evaluation of the risks—but that would not be true. I have no idea why I chose, not only to run into the fire, but to lead many others into it as well. I am not a hero—never have been and never will be—but I am lucky enough to have been surrounded by many heroes during my three decades as a nurse. To all of the social justice warriors who led me down this path— my mom, dad, and siblings; Jim and Sam; Boston's gay community; the many patients from MGH and their journeys through life and death; my friends and mentors in ANAC; and all the PIH staff around the world—thank you for showing me the way.

SUPPLEMENTAL RESOURCES

- MGH Institute of Health Professions
  www.mghihp.edu
- Northeastern University co-op program
  https://bouve.northeastern.edu/nursing/programs
- The ANAC website has the best resources that are kept up to date
  https://www.nursesinaidscare.org/i4a/pages/index.cfm?pageid=4684
- Association of Nurses in AIDS Care (ANAC)
  www.nursesinaidscare.org
- Massachusetts General Hospital Infectious Diseases Unit
  https://www.massgeneral.org/infectiousdisease
- Partners In Health (PIH)
  www.pih.org

Forging a Different Path at the Intersection of Nursing and Innovation

KELLY LARRABEE-ROBKE, MBA, MS, BSN, RN

> *"Two roads diverged in a wood, and I—I took the one less traveled by, and that has made all the difference."*
>
> —Robert Frost

Nursing has afforded me the most challenging, rewarding, and amazing career. From inpatient to high-risk obstetrics, labor and delivery, and oncology (melanoma), I have worked in a variety of units in so many different settings. Through nursing, I have also been able to observe how many of my colleagues poured their hearts and souls into their patients' health. I have seen how much patients rely on the services of nursing and personally understand that we, as nurses, have the power to engage and evolve healthcare as leaders, which has long been my call to action. This road has always led to the patient, but there are many paths that allow you to impact that moment, that care delivery episode, that hospital, that nurse, in a variety of different ways.

I started down the path of nursing as a staff nurse in high-risk obstetrics. The fascinating part of this role was the challenge of two patients: a mother and her baby. Integrating data from both helps to ensure adequate outcomes; the use of technology in this space was, and is, essential in ensuring the safety of mother and baby during the peripartum period. The role of data and its value to care led me to pursue a position as a research nurse, which allowed me to focus on data, innovation, and how outcomes are influenced by novel areas of development in care: through technology, through investigational pharmaceutical medications, and through the observation of the use of existing products in different ways. This led to further career opportunities in pharmaceutical and medical device companies, and research of operational groups that deliver innovative care solutions to the healthcare industry.

Success in these parallel and complementary paths afforded me the opportunity to expand the boundaries of my career path, through positions that developed my clinical, data, and research skills with traditional leadership capabilities. Managing people (both clinicians and nonclinicians) engaged in the delivery of healthcare projects, budgeting, business case development, regulatory engagement, and customer account management are a few examples of the challenges faced in these positions. These opportunities also allowed me to reflect on the value of nursing within industry models of care delivery support systems. The prospect of supporting patient outcomes that impact multiple patients, multiple care environments, and multiple nurses striving to deliver this care was a motivating factor to continue traveling this career route.

As I reflect on this nontraditional journey, I can proudly say that much of my achievement stems from the generosity and dedication that others have poured into enabling my success.

From my grandmother, an immigrant who believed I could do anything enough for the both of us, to my uncle, who taught me the value of education, I was provided with the groundwork to academically and professionally recognize success. My parents also both afforded me the benefit of work ethic and commitment to a job well done, setting the bar for my high-achiever status in life. And I cannot forget the nurses I have worked with, the many lifelong friends, who have supported and encouraged me when I didn't see my own abilities. Some of these people include my college roommates, such great women and nurses, who gave me the framework to find my groove in becoming a nurse. These two amazing clinicians still afford me with that support and insight even today. With this amazing village, I can truly say I have been fortunate enough to benefit from family support and amazing mentors, and been lucky enough to know myself, to take risks, and learn from challenges in a manner that has built resiliency and determination.

In addition to the support from those around me, my mentors have also been so generous with their experience and insights, which provided me with opportunities to succeed, and permission to fail, in endeavors that ultimately served as growth opportunities in my career. In my opinion, mentors are invaluable. However, I have also learned that to be truly innovative, it may be worth choosing mentors in alternative roles beyond nursing, in addition to those you may find in the nursing profession. Also, when searching for a mentor, consider looking for those who will both nurture and challenge you in your abilities, opinions, and approaches. Ideally, they should have once walked along the road less traveled, too.

For me, some memorable mentors in my career were the physician fellows I worked with when I was a research nurse, who believed in me and saw me as an equal, not a subordinate, and who instilled the value of contributing to the overarching body of healthcare knowledge that can be used to deliver care improvements now and over time. These incredible leaders also included many other non-nursing professionals, such as pharmacists, medical technologists, physicians, and information technology executives. They all saw the value in me as a nurse, and in the practice of nursing, in achieving health and well-being for patients.

Another lesson that I have learned is that in keeping an open mind, and identifying my true passions—for research, for improvements, for caring, for technology—I have forged a path that not even I could have imagined. I have been offered opportunities in healthcare operations, information technology, clinical research, and project management that have allowed me to impact healthcare delivery, nursing practice, and innovation on a global scale to the benefit of nursing and patient populations, beyond the individualized point of care. These passions outside nursing also pushed me to pursue a nontraditional degree in finance, strategy, and operations, which gave me the benefit of balancing clinical knowledge with business acumen. My MBA allowed me to be considered for nonclinical roles in the healthcare industry that needed a resource who could represent the needs of the business, in addition to the insights of clinical care delivery. Business and clinical acumen also afford a unique and compelling skill set that helps recognize innovative opportunities and alternatives to approaching business and care delivery, which may not be inherently possible when focusing on them separately. In speaking both of these languages while walking my path, I have been allowed to continue to expand my efforts in acting as a voice of empowerment for nursing, and therefore for patients.

It most instrumentally led me to work within the BD Medication Management Division for 6 years, having been hired into a product management leadership role for Pyxis Medstation by one of my now-mentors, a pharmacist. As over 1.3 million RNs use Pyxis every day in care delivery, the vision of nursing in enterprise medication management is not only desirable, but necessary. Soliciting relevant product feedback, incorporating this into our product development life cycle, and weighing the delivery of a variety of features with the long-term vision of our product portfolio were responsibilities that did not always require me to lead with clinical skills; but, my passion for nursing was evident in the outputs of our enterprise product evolution journey. Along with an amazing group of colleagues from product, R&D (research and development), implementation, and commercialization, we were able to introduce the second generation of Pyxis that serviced healthcare customers from an enterprise technology perspective. This collaborative design of the second generation Pyxis ultimately led to: the incorporating of relevant guidelines and prompts into workflows involving patient assignments; creating a more convenient system for documenting work activity, at the actual point of an activity (such as witnessing a narcotic waste); as well as streamlining the time-consuming efforts that nurses needed to exert during narcotic counts that occurred at shift change. In working in this role, I was able to grow skills in strategic planning, and have been promoted as a result of the successes recognized through teamwork and belief in our efforts to transform medication management.

My current position as Vice President of Clinical Thought Leadership allows me to lead organization efforts to engage clinicians in supporting key opinion leader knowledge sharing, innovation, and driving clinician involvement in product development. This role involves managing our network of clinician advisors, working with our business units on incorporating clinician feedback into product design and commercialization efforts, delivering novel customer engagement opportunities like hackathons and innovation labs, and expanding our continuing education course offerings to our clinician community. We also develop channels for nurses to deliver presentations and share valuable information with colleagues at a variety of national and global conferences.

As a nurse, I still rely upon my role assigned to me 29 years ago to act as a leader in healthcare delivery, and as an advocate for patients and clinicians alike. And because I have had my road in healthcare paved by the determination and generosity of many people, I am now using it to build a path for others who are coming up along the road less traveled. I am now using my influence to build a path for others who may need my unique support. To all the amazing caregivers who forged the path that helped me thrive and achieve: the nurses with whom I worked with on various units, the customers who shared their insights and challenges with me, and the nursing thought leaders with whom I am honored to work with today—I am deeply appreciative. Because of them, I am driven to continue to pay-it-forward to others. So now, as I continue to trail blaze and challenge the status quo to the benefit of nursing, I am committed to supporting others as they walk down new roads that they will forge as the rebel nurses of the future.

SUPPLEMENTAL RESOURCES

- BD Medication Management Division
  https://www.bd.com/en-in/our-products/medication-management
- Broome, M. E., & Marshall, E. S. (2021). *Transformational leadership in nursing: From expert clinician to influential leader*, (3rd ed.). New York, NY: Springer Publishing Company.

What the Hack?! How a Nursing Hackathon Changed My Career

CHRISTINE M. O'BRIEN, DNP, MSHI, RN-BC, FIEL

"Failure will take you to success, if you learn from it. If you can learn from it, it will be the ultimate pivot point in your journey."

Dan Feinberg, EdD, MBA

Throughout our careers, we are faced with numerous decisions to make about professional development. We pursue opportunities sometimes as part of a master plan and sometimes as an ad hoc prospect. My personal experience, as it is for many medical professionals, is a blend of both—a well-thought-out path, and unique opportunities that have presented themselves along life's journey. I reached a career inflection point in 2017, and a series of opportunities and decisions led my career in a direction that I had not previously conceived.

In June 2017, Northeastern University, my alma mater, held its first ever nursing hackathon, a 3-day event for nurses to create and cultivate solutions to today's healthcare delivery challenges. This event, while sponsored and delivered by the university, was developed and orchestrated by nurses. Overwhelmingly popular with the local nursing community, the hackathon provided an outlet for nurses to engineer solutions in the form of applications, devices, and programs. It ultimately developed their previously undiscovered entrepreneurial spirit.

Fast forward a few years, and I find that my participation in the nursing hackathon provided me something not advertised in the brochure—unbounded confidence in myself. I've found that sometimes our most influential events come out of the blue, not researched, not planned, not anticipated; they just happen. The hackathon was one of those events for me. It ultimately put me on a career trajectory that, frankly, was beyond my wildest professional dreams. It's amazing what a little self-awakening can do for our spirit and motivation.

When a colleague and friend approached me about the hackathon, I was working as an informatics nurse at an academic medical center. I had been in the nursing field for 20 years and enjoyed a very full range of experiences at work. When I graduated from nursing school, I had no idea about informatics. At the time it was not a course, much less an advertised career path. Over the past decade, I have met many nurses in informatics who share that experience. It was not a field that we actively pursued, but more of an opportunity presented to us that made professional sense. I became a nursing informaticist through a series of fortunate events. At the time, I may have interpreted these events as challenges, but now I see them clearly as catalysts for positive change.

When I first graduated from nursing school, I was hired by the academic medical center where I worked as a nursing student. I worked in a variety of clinical settings, but for the majority of my nursing career I worked as a staff nurse in an adult critical care unit. The intensity of the work and the potential to facilitate positive patient outcomes drove me to always do my best for the patients. I look upon my time in the surgical intensive care unit (SICU) as a major highlight in my career and the scene setter for my future experiences. My work there, my close working relationship with top medical professionals, and my interactions with patients and families forged my composite skill set and formulated my critical thinking. This experience positively impacts my work to this day.

After working in the SICU for 10 years, I had become an experienced professional nurse, well-respected by the medical staff, and delivering the type of care to patients I would want my family to receive. In the midst of this success, I experienced a work-related back injury that forced me off the unit and into a less physically intensive role at the hospital. As I reflect back now, the physical pain and professional disruption was difficult to manage at the time. However, I now know this was part of my personal and professional process to create new opportunities for growth and achievement. At the time of my injury, the hospital was introducing a new barcode medication administration (BMA) system. I was invited to join this start-up, and get in on the ground floor as the hospital embraced the growth of healthcare information technology (IT). I consider myself to be very fortunate to have joined the superuser group that helped support this new IT initiative.

My new team trained nearly every nurse on the BMA system. While some of the technical aspects could be tedious at times, I found the opportunity broadly fulfilling in that I took great pride and enjoyment in helping my colleagues become more adept as nurses. Having overcome my medical challenge, and infused with a new sense of optimism and purpose, I decided to make informatics my next career move. I applied for and accepted a permanent position in the nursing informatics department. Working in this department opened my eyes to the vastness of technology's application in the medical field. While I learned about all the various components of the IT infrastructure, I was particularly interested in healthcare IT adoption and the system development life cycle. Through experiential activities I was able to hone and ultimately perfect my project management skills. As an empowered informaticist, I was inspired by my capacity to effect change throughout the entire institution. I cherished the role of being able to support clinicians in helping them deliver the best possible care to patients. With this new sense of purpose, I enrolled in a master of health informatics program at Northeastern.

Seven years into my informatics career, I was well on track and proceeding in a logical and predictable manner. As what would become a welcome disruption, my director proposed that I attend a nursing hackathon as a representative of the medical center. Truthfully, neither of us knew exactly what a nursing hackathon was, but we were nurses and we inferred the "hacking" had something to do with computers, so we thought we had to go and check this out! Intrigued, my colleague and I registered for the program.

Having done some background research on the nature of these hackathons, I entered the ballroom on a Friday evening and still can recall the excitement generated by the participants. After listening to great presentations from a range of nursing professionals and entrepreneurs for inspiration, it was time to pitch ideas. More than 20 nurses presented amazing ideas on how to improve healthcare delivery. Following the structure of the hackathon, I had to select one of the pitches that resonated with me and join their team. After much deliberation, I joined a team aiming to identify, through social media, people who were sick. The pitch was a social media app that would identify that "Jane" had flu symptoms 1 day ago, and had to inform her friends and family of the potential micro and macro impacts that would have on society. For example, we would not be eating Jane's homemade appetizers at the holiday party if we knew she was sick yesterday. After robust and far-flung discussions, team members strategized for an hour.

Early Saturday morning, we met up in a conference room on campus and got to work. With laptops in hand, we made use of a smartboard and a dry erase board, conceptualizing who might be users of this idea. Throughout the day, we brainstormed and talked through different ideas with experienced mentors. These mentors (think Project Runway's Tim Gunn) rotated in and out of the room offering us feedback and asking probing questions that caused us to pivot to a different direction. When we set aside our egos and preconceived notions, and accepted constructive criticism, our idea crystallized and really took off. At the end of the day, our idea went into a completely new direction as a bolt-on application that would work in conjunction with a school system application to assist school nurses in tracking students' illnesses.

We returned early that Sunday morning for the big "Shark Tank" moment. The teams presented their final products. I was really pleasantly stunned and blown away by how far the teams developed their ideas in less than 48 hours. That afternoon, the big moment arrived, and we were thrilled to find out that our project placed second out of nine teams. While winning is always a fun event, we were very satisfied and proud to have achieved so much in such a short time.

When the high-fives, cheers, and smiles were done, we experienced the "now what" moment. Fortunately for us, our prize included a business 101 class for nurses. The course helped us navigate the next steps: purchasing the domain name, securing the company name, deciding which type of corporate structure would be best, formulating a business plan, creating a market analysis, and many other relevant topics. Furthermore, our second-place prize also offered us a luncheon with leadership from an investment firm. The CEO offered us some great advice that was relevant and insightful. My biggest takeaway was to never underestimate our nursing knowledge and experience. The CEO told us that companies would be willing to pay for the experience and intelligence we as nurses already possess. Unfortunately, as is often the case in the business world, our team was never able to get the project to the finish line. It was a great idea but ultimately, we were unable to gain traction with the implementation of the concept.

Gladly, my story does not end there, as the whole experience became an inflection point for my career. As deflating as the demise of our project was, the process was a transformative event that inspired me to create new opportunities for myself and ultimately re-engineer my career. I pursued a leadership position and went on to obtain my DNP degree. I attribute these achievements, in part, to the inspiring and enlightened individuals who came into my life as a result of that monumental weekend.

One of my health informatics professors, Dan Feinberg, EdD, MBA, had told me, "Failure will take you to success, if you learn from it. If you can learn from it, it will be the ultimate pivot point in your journey." The hackathon experience changed me. It altered my perception and clarified my view of reality. I discovered a world that I didn't know existed for me as a nurse.

SUPPLEMENTAL RESOURCES

- Northeastern University, Bouvé School of Nursing
  https://bouve.northeastern.edu/nursing
- Khoury College of Computer Sciences, Health Informatics
  https://www.khoury.northeastern.edu/program/health-informatics-ms
- Hardy, L. R. (2020). *Fast facts in health informatics for nurses.* New York, NY: Springer Publishing Company.
- McBride, S., & Tietze, M. *Nursing informatics for the advanced practice nurse: Patient safety, quality, outcomes, and interprofessionalism,* (2nd ed.). New York, NY: Springer Publishing Company.

Living a Life by Design

JOANNA SELTZER URIBE, MSN, RN, EdD

"I AM INSPIRED TO ENCOURAGE OTHER NURSES TO BROADEN THE DEFINITION OF WHAT NURSES ARE CAPABLE OF. THEIR INSIGHTS AND IDEAS CAN CREATE MEANINGFUL CONTRIBUTIONS TO THE FUTURE OF HEALTHCARE."

From the youngest age, my connection to the world around me was never theoretical. As an 8- or 9-year-old drawing with chalk on the sidewalk, I would inscribe neighborly reminders of "give a hoot, don't pollute" and "reduce, reuse, and recycle." A few years later, my neighbor and I sold Valentine's cookies and gave the proceeds to Greenpeace. A few years after that, my friends and I transformed a forgotten triangle of dirt at an intersection in my town with tulips as an HIV/AIDS memorial garden.

I was an avid dancer from ages 8 to 18. Between requisite suburban Nutcracker dance performances, I choreographed a piece at my middle school about the experience of being an adolescent during the war in Bosnia. By my early twenties, I was protesting the Gulf War with my family in DC. Maybe it was the steady stream of NPR during dinner, hearing John Lennon's "Imagine" on repeat, or simply my own naivete, but I've always felt connected to causes for humanity and planet Earth—somehow steadfastly certain at a young age that humans were capable of positively impacting the world if we only set our minds to it.

A knee injury made me reconsider pursuing dancing as a young adult, so I detoured into liberal arts and was introduced to anatomy, physiology, and farming in the same semester. Farming taught me everything that I had missed while spending my summers in dance studios and it connected me to the source of our food and nourishment, which growing up in the suburbs did not afford. Learning about my own anatomy, quite frankly, was mind-blowing. As a dancer, the curriculum is in the movement itself, but anatomy was a new world opened to me from a single—and mammoth—textbook. I was hooked and, soon after, decided the best way to find out more about this body I call home was to apply to nursing school.

Like many nursing grads before me and those after me, I began on the night shift in a medical/surgical unit of a busy urban hospital. Feeling that I needed more exposure to specialties, I ultimately joined a travel nurse organization and was assigned to a kidney transplant department. This move showed me a whole new side of healthcare, one in which patients, after their transplants, were *getting better*—their health and quality of life were improving. The majority of care was provided in an outpatient setting, rather than inpatient. The classical paradigm of a nurse physically administering medication to patients according to schedule shifted to calling in prescriptions for patients, and thereafter calling them with instructions as they resumed their more independent life off dialysis.

However, there was a glaring aspect of kidney transplantation that made little sense to me—the amount of paper charts *everywhere*. The sheer management of storing charts, finding charts, and updating charts was a job in and of itself. At best, we found what we needed without much delay; at worst, patients would wait to be seen until we could locate their chart, and their care was delayed until we could find the medication list or the last physician's note. Some charts, having been utilized for years of the patient's care, were so full that there were two separate volumes for the same patient! As a transplant nurse coordinator, I had a front row seat in experiencing the shift from paper to electronic medical records—and it was not pretty.

While the promise of returning the countless staffing hours previously spent maintaining paper charts and flowsheets back to our day should have been celebrated, the electronic medical records were not customized to the needs of such a specialty service. The manual labor spent maintaining the paper charts and flowsheets allowed the staff to contain a vast amount of critical patient data in a centralized place, often on a single, routinely updated, page of the chart. When we transitioned to electronic medical records, there were data fields that didn't exist where we needed to record a patient's last rejection episode, details about patients' medications at the time of their surgery, or critical information about their donor's kidney. We couldn't easily run reports for what we needed in our daily workflows, and since the outpatient electronic medical record was different from the inpatient record, we were needing to constantly log in and out of multiple systems to accurately capture the patient's full picture.

Finding myself as a practicing nurse in the midst of what should have been making our process easier, became my motivation to pursue a graduate degree in nursing informatics. Still an emerging field a decade later, informatics is essentially based on how to meet the needs of providers and patients using healthcare data and information technology. From this perspective, my last decade of working in healthcare has been very multifaceted, as it has been spent in equal parts in direct patient care and in operation, informatics, and quality. My most recent project involved working with a six-person team to transition a kidney transplant department from paper to electronic medical records in 9 months. The project touched outpatient, inpatient, emergency, operating room, laboratory, and imaging departments. The workflows, note templates, order sets, reports, and nurse coordinator checklists we created from scratch are still in use to this day.

What I learned the most by being on the implementation side of electronic medical records is less about the nature of the technology itself, and more on its dependencies on the human element to create its value. This insight, discovered within just a few months upon my graduation, led me to pursue my next field of study: user experience, design thinking, and human-centered design. After attending a design thinking master's series at Stanford's design school, I began to participate in design challenges and, in 2013, as the only nurse on the team, contributed toward a winning finalist proposal for Open IDEO's "How might we all maintain wellbeing and thrive as we age?" global challenge. Looking to bring what I was learning back to informatics students, my nursing informatics director at New York University agreed to let me introduce these concepts to current students in a course called "Designing for Care and Wellness," in which we spend a semester taking students through a design thinking process as a way to augment their informatics pedagogy with a human-centered approach to problem-solving.

In 2018, my work with the New York University nursing graduate students created an opportunity to participate as the lead design thinking expert in an Alex and Rita Hillman–funded grant to introduce design thinking to undergraduate nurses. Our approach was to embed design thinking over 4 semesters uniquely into each course, and I developed new content for both students and faculty that described the design thinking process alongside the nursing process. In a first semester Professional Nursing course, we created several initiatives, including reframing failure (a challenge in the "zero fail" industry of healthcare) and the use of interactive online modules on "Designing Your Life," created by our instructional technologist. Next, we integrated "How Might We...." question definition into the undergraduate research course to demonstrate the path between evidence and research into ideation and action. And we are currently developing the structure for interdisciplinary ideation with students from other New York University schools to tackle social determinants of health. This work has also led to developing and leading several faculty development workshops to introduce design thinking and its concepts of "learning by doing" to nursing educators.

One of the principles of design thinking is centered on "failing forward," which is essentially not allowing a fear of failure to prohibit someone from trying something new and, secondarily, if one's idea or project should "fail," how to extract the maximum insight to improve a process or product going forward. In teaching nursing students to overcome the fear of failure in order to contribute new ideas for their design thinking course assignments, I found myself becoming somewhat of a failure evangelist. In my years as an adjunct professor, I more bravely took on projects outside nursing and nursing informatics. I started a podcast and helped to organize a design week in my town. And, I befriended people outside healthcare through volunteering at conferences and completing training to become a yoga instructor. I also began to view the centralized, traditional idea that healthcare occurs from a hospital bed as one that contributes to myopic solutions in the healthcare space. It is in dire need of revision if we are to ensure that the expertise of nurses is best leveraged across the healthcare ecosystem.

Another concept I was introduced to through my work in design was that of collaboration. Because nursing is intended to be designed as a 'team sport,' one would think today's nurse would know all about collaboration. While true, I would argue that many nurses routinely see what collaboration is *not*. It wasn't until I experienced true collaborators in informatics and design communities that I began to see how the hierarchical nature of healthcare roles can diminish the capacity to leverage collaborative insight. In my 4 years as an informaticist involved with quality improvement, I saw time and again how meetings might center on solutions based on surgeons and physicians and later, in a hallway or behind closed doors, nurses would be more comfortable to speak up with ideas or insights of their own. So after spending over a decade answering my first sets of questions: How does the body work? (nursing degree), how does technology work in healthcare? (informatics degree), and how can design improve healthcare technology? (user experience and human-centered design certificates); I continued to find only more questions—this time around *team-based human behavior*. So this year, I began an interdisciplinary doctorate in education in organizational change to have the opportunity to research questions surrounding culture, collaboration, and fear of failure, and their impact on nursing innovation.

As I am approaching 40 years old, I could feel as though my career is already half over, but instead I feel energized. I have truly just begun to decipher the alchemy between my diverse paths and how they have formed a new, unique perspective. As I expand my areas of research and practice, I look forward to scaling my work in empowering nurses to develop their creative confidence. I am inspired to encourage other nurses to broaden the definition of what nurses are capable of. Their insights and ideas can create meaningful contributions to the future of healthcare.

SUPPLEMENTAL RESOURCES

- The Hasso Plattner Institute of Design at Stanford (d.School)
  https://dschool.stanford.edu
- Open IDEO's "How might we all maintain wellbeing and thrive as we age?" global challenge
  https://challenges.openideo.com/challenge/mayo-clinic/brief
- Designing for Care and Wellness (NYU)
  https://wp.nyu.edu/nursing-consumers
- The Rita and Alex Hillman Foundation
  http://www.rahf.org
- McBride, S., & Tietze, M. *Nursing informatics for the advanced practice nurse: Patient safety, quality, outcomes, and interprofessionalism* (2nd ed.). New York, NY: Springer Publishing Company.
- Sipes, C. (2019). *Application of nursing informatics: Competencies, skills, and decision-making.* New York, NY: Springer Publishing Company

---

In Good Company

KEVIN WHITNEY, DNP, RN, NEA-BC

"INFLUENCE AND INSPIRATION ON THE PATH TO NURSING LEADERSHIP."

As early as I can remember, my dad—a vice president of administration for papermaking by day and call firefighter/emergency medical technician (EMT) by night—was running out the door responding to those in need. Whether a structure fire, brush fire, a person experiencing shortness of breath, or a motor vehicle crash with entrapment, my dad and his call firefighter colleagues responded without hesitation. He quickly emerged as a leader, in large part due to his ability to remain calm in challenging situations and make sound decisions under pressure. His first role as an officer was lieutenant. A few years later, he became a captain until he retired from the fire service. "Captain Dad" (as we called him) soon had another firefighter/ EMT colleague from our family—*my mom*. Mom was the first female firefighter/EMT in our town. She was a trailblazer. Back then, her decision pushed many boundaries, and looking back, I remember not everyone being on board with her decision to enter what was, at the time, a predominantly male profession. However, she was determined, driven, and quickly demonstrated she was extremely capable and successful.

The fire service/emergency medical service (EMS) was a big part of our lives growing up. Watching our parents as they served in their "part-time" profession and witnessing their passion for this role strongly influenced my and my brother's decision to join the department. In our town, you could join the department at age 16 if you had parental permission. Since both our parents were in the department, permission was not a problem. At age 16, and after recruit and first responder training, we were soon responding to fires and medical/trauma emergencies—alongside mom and dad. While my brother focused more on fire prevention and suppression, I was always drawn more to the EMS side of the equation.

My family's story highlights the impact of influence, leadership, mentorship, and taking risks. My parents' influence was powerful. They exposed my brother and me to the fire service, prehospital care, and the rewards and challenges of both roles. They were leaders in their community and role-modeled responsibility. They provided us the opportunity early in life to learn how to cope and manage stressful and emergency situations. They taught us the importance of a strong work ethic and the need for ongoing education and training. They taught us that any gender can perform any role. And most importantly, they taught us the importance of caring and giving back to others in their time of need. To all the nurses reading this—does this sound familiar?

It is no doubt that my upbringing helped shape my decision to enter healthcare over 30 years ago, first as an EMT-paramedic. I attended Northeastern University's EMT-paramedic associate degree program. In addition to completing many clinical rotations in hospitals in the Boston area, I completed my paramedic field internship with New York City EMS (now part of the Fire Department of New York City) in Kings County, Brooklyn. Having passed the National Registry Paramedic written and practical exams, I worked for a private ambulance company for 2 years before landing a highly desired job as a hospital-based paramedic at Emerson Hospital in Concord, MA. Being hired as a paramedic at Emerson was life-changing and added to the impact of my parents' roles, as well as my joining the fire department at a young age, in shaping my future.

As a paramedic at Emerson, we provided advanced life support care to the 14 surrounding communities in collaboration with each town fire department. Between 911 calls, we worked in the ED and assisted the RNs, physicians, and ED technicians with patient care, including starting intravenous (IV) lines, administering medications, and responding to codes. It was also at Emerson where I met my wife of 28 years, Cindy, an ED RN at that time. The year after we were married, I was strongly considering returning to school to obtain my bachelor's degree. I knew I wanted to remain in healthcare and thought about several health profession disciplines. Cindy said, "Why don't you become an RN … you can do many things as a nurse … different specialties, education, or leadership." It was excellent advice. Looking back, I am grateful that I listened.

Just as my dad supported my mom's decision to become a firefighter/EMT, Cindy supported 100% my return to school to obtain my BSN and enter into practice as an RN. I attended the University of Massachusetts-Lowell full-time for 3½ years, while continuing to work full-time as a paramedic. We also had just built a home, and during my first semester back to school, our daughter, Kerri, was born. During my junior year our son, Zach, was born. Kerri was born during spring break and Zach over Columbus Day weekend—I didn't miss a class. All kidding aside, it was a busy time (and sometimes stressful), but it was worth it. However, it wouldn't have been possible without Cindy and her incredible support.

After passing the RN boards, I first worked in the ICU. Given my paramedic background and exposure to working in the ED while going to school, however, I knew my clinical home was the ED. I transitioned to the ED as an RN, where I spent most of my full-time direct-care career. While working in the ED, a colleague decided to work per diem after accepting a job in clinical research, managing pharmaceutical and medical device trials. I was intrigued by this role, and after learning more, I applied and entered industry while continuing to work part time in the ED.

I first worked for a contract research organization, and then was recruited to a large medical device/health care products company. As a clinical research associate, I primarily coordinated postmarketing trials and user preference testing, as well as supported 510k submissions, which are technical documents created to show a product's safety and effectiveness, for Food and Drug Administration (FDA) approvals (U.S. Food and Drug Administration, 2018). One of my first experiences with innovation was working with the research and development team refining a prototype of a safety hypodermic needle, the Monoject Magellan. This safety needle device required clinicians to passively activate a safety sheath over the needle after use.

To obtain FDA 510k approval, we conducted simulated use testing to demonstrate that the needle could be used safely by clinicians, was intuitive, could be activated only using one hand, and was reliable. I was responsible for coordinating three sites to conduct the simulated use testing, writing the simulation use protocol, and creating the data collection forms. We worked with a statistician to review data collected and demonstrated a 99% confidence interval that the needle could be used safely and without failure.

I was the lead author of a white paper for the product and presented a poster at the Association for Practitioners of Infection Control (APIC) National Conference in Nashville, TN. It was an awesome experience; however, I was navigating in uncharted waters, as I had not coordinated this type of testing previously. This project allowed me the opportunity to learn by researching the FDA regulations and guidance documents, and be mentored by my engineering and regulatory colleagues. It also highlighted the importance of nurses being involved in informing product design and other innovations. Nurses play a key role as part of the design team, and it is important to ensure nursing's voice is at the table.

After 3 years working full time in industry and enhancing my leadership skills while continuing to work in the ED part time, I had the opportunity to combine both skill sets and returned to the ED full time as an associate nurse manager. I believe the exposure to strong nursing leaders contributed to my interest in becoming a leader, and has helped shape the leader I am today and continue to strive to be.

A key nursing leadership mentor, Linda Wells, MBA, RN, was the vice president of patient care services and chief nursing officer (CNO) at Emerson Hospital. Linda was very inspiring, charismatic, patient-centered, and staff-focused, as well as collaborative, respectful, and trustworthy. She modeled how a leader can positively influence and motivate others to action. Linda offered me my first department-level leadership role of nurse manager of the ED, promoting me from my associate nurse manager role. She frequently asked me to lead various projects from the design phase through implementation and evaluation. Over time, she increased my scope of responsibility by adding two additional departments. Over a 6-year period, she continued to offer roles with progressively more responsibility, including a promotion to director of inpatient services.

A second key mentor, Jeanette Ives Erickson, DNP, RN, FAAN, chief nurse emeritus at Massachusetts General Hospital (MGH), held many of the same characteristics. Like Linda, she was a very strategic, visionary, and innovative leader. She developed the innovation unit effort at MGH, where inpatient units trialed tests of change to improve the quality of care and experience along the patient journey. Under her leadership, the entire care team created a bundle of interventions designed to "manage between the spaces" along the patient care journey (prior to admission, during admission, preparing for discharge, and postdischarge).

One of the interventions was a new nursing role on each unit called the "attending nurse," who helped coordinate the patient's care in partnership with the patient's primary nurse and other members of the care team. During the innovation unit effort, there were interventions within the bundle that were very effective (attending nurse) and others less effective. "Adopt, adapt, or abandon" was Jeanette's mantra, which helped the team feel empowered to adopt an intervention as designed, modify one that needed tweaking, and abandon those that were not providing the desired outcome or workflow.

I witnessed the positive impact both Linda and Jeanette had on patient care, patient satisfaction, staff engagement, and the professional work environment. Both are caring and emotionally intelligent leaders whom I sincerely admire. I am grateful for all the life experiences and the "wise advice" that led me to the decision to become an RN and later a doctorally prepared nurse leader. It takes hard work, but if you are determined and driven, you can achieve any goal. Whether you are entering nursing or advancing your education within the profession, I offer the following advice and words of support:

- If you put your mind to something, along with the influence and support from family, friends, and colleagues, you can do anything.

- Find a mentor who can help inspire and advance your clinical and leadership practice.

- Don't be afraid to take risks. It is okay to "adapt" or "abandon" if necessary.

- You have many opportunities as a nurse ... direct care provider, educator, formal leader, researcher, innovator, entrepreneur—be courageous.

- Be a trailblazer!

SUPPLEMENTAL RESOURCES

- National Registry of Emergency Medical Technicians
  https://www.nremt.org/rwd/public
- University of Massachusetts Lowell
  https://www.uml.edu
- Association for Practitioners of Infection Control (APIC) National Conference
  https://apic.org
  https://ac2019.site.apic.org
- Emerson Hospital
  https://www.emersonhospital.org
- Mass General Nursing Innovation Enters New Era
  https://giving.massgeneral.org/nursing-innovation-enters-new-era
- Premarket Notification 510(k)
  https://www.fda.gov/medical-devices/premarket-submissions/premarket-notification-510k

Take the Risk; Fortune Favors the Bold

BRIAN WEIRICH, DHA, MHA, BSN, CENP

"*My goal here is to create a vision and use evidence-based medicine and innovation to challenge the status quo and begin doing my part in leading changes in healthcare.*"

A week before prom during my junior year of high school, I was sitting in the bleachers at our local fairgrounds watching a "mock crash" drunk driving scene play out in front of me. First, I heard the blades in the distance, and then the helicopter came into view and landed on the field. As the nurse and medic jumped out in their suits to "rescue the victim," I decided then and there, I wanted to be a nurse, specifically a flight nurse.

After graduating with my associate's degree in nursing, my first role was as an RN in the medical intensive care unit at the Cleveland Clinic. I learned a lot of essential clinical and leadership skills during my time at the Clinic. I experienced the highs and lows of health-care, as well as teamwork, the importance of being dependable, and finding a support system. However, it wasn't long before I moved to Columbus, Ohio, and took a staff nurse position in an open heart ICU at The Ohio State Medical Center where I had previously been a nurse aide before nursing school. After a few years, I quickly realized there are "size requirements" for flight nurses that would make my entry into this field difficult, if not impossible.

Later in my career, the following quote by Phil Knight, the co-founder of Nike, Inc., became vital to me; it resonates with me as I reflect on several instances throughout my career—never more prevalent than when I asked myself "what now?" for the first time after deciding to pursue something other than flight nursing. I'm proud to be a nurse, but I wanted to make a difference on a bigger scale. I wanted to "put a dent in the universe", as Steve Jobs often said.

"*Deep down, I was searching for something else, something more. I had this aching sense that our time is short, shorter than we ever know, short as a morning run, and I wanted mine to be meaningful. And purposeful. And creative. And important. Above all . . . different. I wanted to leave a mark on the world.*"

— *Phil Knight, Shoe Dog, p. 3*

I wasn't sure how to do this but knew that leadership would be the best path. I would have a more substantial influence and greater decision-making ability. Within a month, I began pursuing my bachelor's degree in nursing and accepted my first assistant manager job in the acute dialysis unit at The Ohio State Medical Center. Although I was not familiar with hemo-dialysis, I was eager to develop as a leader in the environment and in the role. In my years at Ohio State, I also completed my BSN and my master's in healthcare administration (MHA) at Ohio University. Through my many roles with larger scopes, I eventually ended up as a manager in the perioperative arena.

Working my way up the ladder, I accepted a leadership position in oncology at Barnes Jewish Hospital in St. Louis, MO. From there, I found myself in a director role at the University of Colorado Health with oversight over service lines at hospitals in Loveland

and Fort Collins. Here I began expanding my leadership and influence beyond the hospital walls, making a more substantial impact on the nursing profession and the healthcare industry.

I became a member of the inaugural director fellow cohort of the American Organization of Nurse Executives (AONE), as well as a committee board member for the state chapter Colorado Organization of Nurse Leaders. On behalf of these organizations, I spent time on Capitol Hill lobbying for issues that impacted our patients and clinicians. This experience would serve me well in the years to follow.

Around this same time, the millennial workforce began to grow exponentially in numbers. There was an overwhelmingly negative perspective of these workers. They were described as: "narcissistic," "self-interested," "unfocused," and "lazy." As a millennial who does not fit into these common biases, I took it as my role to change the conversation on a global scale. In contrast to the negative perception that many people have of millennials, this group of workers who grew up in the *tech age* are perfectly suited for the current fast-paced environment we work in today. In my articles, I published my thoughts: "A Millennial Leader's Views on the Millennial Workforce," published in *Nurse Leader* magazine, and "How Millennial Leaders in the Healthcare Industry Can Uniquely Contribute and Thrive," published in *Becker's Hospital Review*. In 2016, I decided to launch a podcast called "The Report Room: A Podcast for Nurses and Nurse Leaders. Itunes published 12 episodes, including such topics as patient stories, nurse stories, and CEO pathways. Former Ohio State Buckeye head coach, Jim Tressel, talked leader development, and New Belgium Brewery discussed their unique employee rewards program. This experience gave me the confidence to jump into unfamiliar waters, to learn and find my success.

After completing my doctorate in healthcare administration from The Medical University of South Carolina in 2016, I transitioned into a chief nursing officer role at Indiana University Health, the C-suite. My goal here is to create a vision and use evidence-based medicine and innovation to challenge the status quo, and begin doing my part in leading changes in healthcare. This is easier said than done. With many external pressures and an unknown future, the industry has become intensely risk-averse, and budgets are tight. Dollars are not set aside to "try new things." This was never more obvious to me than when I tried to solve the problem of ED patients leaving without being seen.

Throughput became my nemesis, and reduced hospital flow led to ED holds and patients leaving the ED before a physician could assess them. One of the problems we identified was that when the ED is struggling, no resources come to rescue them. To solve this, we went to the startup world and found a small local company that could develop both the hardware and software for a device that changes color, reflecting the real-time status of the ED on a five-point scale: from normal to dangerously overcrowded. It was not easy. The infrastructure works against such innovations. I was able to get a small donation/grant from the community, and ran a budget variance to cover the remaining few thousand dollars, relatively small expenses for something that has had a tremendous impact. Currently, anywhere you go in the hospital, an LED light reflects the real-time status of the ED.

Over the next 2 years, I became intrigued by artificial intelligence and the role it can and will play in the industry. Using Alexa and Siri is unbelievably efficient and so easy that my children use technology daily. With this task-focused workforce, we need to bring this technology into the hospital for frontline staff to use to navigate large volumes of data in real-time. After talking with Amazon and facing more barriers, I decided to build my own. Learning from previous experiences with new technology and the minimal resources from within, I entered the startup world—this time as an entrepreneur and founder myself. Through this endeavor I developed aRNi™, a combination of artificial intelligence and registered nurse. aRNi is a closed-loop voice assistant that can be customized by healthcare systems, which have total control over what information is given in response to clinician inquiries. As a result of this technology, I was awarded a $150,000 Advancement in Medicine Grant from the Indiana University School of Medicine to pursue this project and bring it to scale.

Recently, I began problem-solving population health and the frequent admissions and readmissions from the chronic patient population. Two things stood out to me: first, literature showing that the aging general population would prefer independence and care at home; and second, a younger workforce who wants to work when they want, where they want, and do what they want. I see this as a perfect fit to utilize crowd-sourcing and the gig economy to address the perceived ambulatory/outpatient clinician shortage. Existing employees could and would "moonlight," i.e., cover these needs if given the opportunity. Hence, the formation of the startup iMoonlite, and again the exhilarating process of funding, building, and executing being put into motion. iMoonlite is a member of the NY-based accelerator StartUp Health's health transformer community.

The quote shared by Chef John Folse, "risk is the tariff paid to leave the shores of predictable misery" recently caught my attention (The Chef's Garden, 2016). In the 11 years since my graduation from nursing school, my journey has been full of risks. I have gone back to school four times and relocated five times throughout four different states. I've sat on state and national boards, and have always been the first to volunteer for large projects. Then, instead of sitting comfortably in the C-suite, I ventured into the startup world. In addition, I am married to a nurse, and we have five small children.

Along with the accomplishments mentioned above, I am a co-author of the book, *The Nurse's Guide to Innovation: Accelerating the Journey,* and I am also a founding member of the Society of Nurse Scientists, Innovators, Entrepreneurs, and Leaders (SONSIEL). Connect with me on twitter @BrianWeirichRN.

SUPPLEMENTAL RESOURCES

- Medical Intensive Care Unit at the Cleveland Clinic
  https://my.clevelandclinic.org
- Open-Heart ICU at The Ohio State Medical Center
  https://wexnermedical.osu.edu
- Barnes Jewish Hospital in St. Louis, MO
  https://www.barnesjewish.org
- University of Colorado Health
  https://www.uchealth.org
- American Organization of Nurse Executives (AONE)
  https://www.aonl.org
- Colorado Organization of Nurse Leaders
  https://www.coloradonurseleaders.org
- A Millennial Leader's Views on the Millennial Workforce, published in *Nurse Leader*
  https://www.nurseleader.com
- How Millennial Leaders in the Healthcare Industry Can Uniquely Contribute and Thrive, published in *Becker's Hospital Review*
  https://www.beckershospitalreview.com/hospital-management-administration/how-millennial-leaders-in-the-healthcare-industry-can-uniquely-contribute-and-thrive.html

- *The Report Room: A podcast for nurses & nurse leaders*
  https://player.fm/series/the-report-room-nursing-professionals-health-care-medical-profession
- New Belgium Brewery: their unique employee rewards program
  https://www.newbelgium.com/brewery/fort-collins
- The Medical University of South Carolina
  https://web.musc.edu
- Indiana University Health
  https://iuhealth.org
- aRNi™
  http://www.creations86.com
- Advancement in Medicine Grant from the Indiana University School of Medicine
  https://medicine.iu.edu
- iMoonlite
  http://imoonlite.com
- StartUp Health's health transformer community
  https://www.startuphealth.com

A Rebel Curriculum

JENNIFER WALLACE, MSN, RN

> *"KNOW THE RULES WELL SO YOU CAN BREAK THEM EFFECTIVELY."*
> —THE DALAI LAMA

Sitting at the family dinner table, I was acutely aware of my racing pulse and sweaty palms. I had been rehearsing this announcement for days and now the time had come to inform our close friends and family that we were planning to homeschool our oldest daughter. It would be the first of many awkward and uncomfortable conversations.

Her year of public school kindergarten had been challenging. Many days had ended with tears and exhaustion. The teacher had expressed concern that our daughter's quiet and somewhat shy personality put her at risk of getting lost in the next year's proposed classroom size of 30 students. My husband and I had done our due diligence. We researched the legalities and logistics, spoke to other homeschooling families, and most importantly confirmed that our daughter was on board. We were fortunate that my per diem position as a staff nurse at a local hospital provided me with not only a paycheck but also flexible hours close to home.

I felt confident about our decision, but was very nervous to break the news. Sitting around that table was a clinical nurse specialist turned public school teacher, a child psychiatrist, a dean of students at a prestigious local university, and a plastic surgeon—people who fiercely loved my daughter, but also placed a high value on formal education. I realized that there would be no easy entry for the news. It would be best to just blurt it out. After it was out, I looked around the table and noticed everyone had stopped chewing and was staring at their plates.

Over the following weeks and months, we broke the news to others in our close circle of friends and family and heard a host of well-meaning, but uninformed concerns, most related to commonly held stereotypes about homeschooling: *What about her socialization? What about the prom? What about college?* My feeble responses reflected how I felt at the time: hesitant, scared, and a bit embarrassed about our plan.

Although I felt secure in our decision to homeschool, I was less confident in the beginning about how we were going to execute it. I approached it as I do most other projects—by giving 100% with a can-do attitude.

Gathering my courage, I reached out to our local public school administration. During an in-person meeting with the curriculum director, I proposed a plan that would allow my daughter to participate in either art, music, or physical education with her same grade peers. Not only did I leave that first meeting with my proposal accepted, I also left with a bag full of books currently in use by the first grades across the district. The director showed me how to use the teacher version and assured me that her door was always open if I had questions. I was elated! In time, my younger daughter joined her sister in homeschooling. Both girls went on to participate in a variety of school and community activities from sports to drama. Through the years, the principals, staff, and teachers were welcoming and encouraging. This positive, early experience was emboldening and marked the start of my interest in alternative education.

We were blessed to have also been a part of a wonderful local grassroots cooperative of homeschooling families. Together, we founded and ran a successful cooperative where children learned in small group settings. Most teachers were parents who spun their professional knowledge and expertise into classes. This co-op also gave older teens the opportunity to develop and teach classes for younger children. When there was an interest in a topic, but no available parent, dues allowed us to hire an outside teacher. The children took classes in math, science, foreign languages, creative writing, cooking, health, knitting, theater, art, and music. Although, the co-op's location changed through the years, we were primarily housed in churches as they were affordable and empty during the week. Through my involvement with the co-op, I experienced the joys of facilitating authentic, student-centered collaborative education. I also learned that many struggles come along with building an infrastructure, allocating scarce resources, and making decision by committee.

During my time homeschooling, I began to wonder what made families choose homeschooling over a traditional educational setting. Through observation and conversations with other parents, I came to understand that many children experience the typical classroom like an ill-fitting shoe. It just doesn't feel right and for some it is downright painful. It may be temperament or a disconnect in learning styles, or for others, like my younger daughter, diagnosed with dyslexia as a junior in high school, the cause may be a learning disability (LD). So for varied reasons, the traditional classroom experience does not sing to the strengths of all students. From this personal interest, came the opportunity to help plan a parent seminar about learning disabilities and homeschooling.

In my current nurse educator role, I recently revisited this long-standing interest. It has been my observation that some students have a great deal of difficulty in the class, but are shining stars in the clinical setting. During conversations in my role as an academic, some of these students have confessed that they struggle to keep up because of reading or attentional issues. The high-stakes nature of testing and the rapid delivery of content has resulted in significant stress and anxiety. As the mother of a child with an LD, I have an intimate understanding of the toxic effects that this can have on a student's physical or emotional health, well-being, and readiness to learn. This past semester, in collaboration with a colleague from the education department, I co-presented a faculty development program about LDs in nursing education. I also attended a 3-day conference the summer of 2019 focusing on universal design in learning (UDL). I believe that this curricular model, very familiar to our colleagues in education, holds promise for helping *all* nursing students access content more successfully—not just those with LDs. This has relevance as we strive to diversify the nursing workforce, and welcome many nontraditional students and students of all abilities into our programs.

Both of my parents were teachers. Unlike some of my students, I have always found school to be an easy fit for me. I have fond memories of being very young and sitting in the back of my father's college classroom, and copying mathematical symbols from the board into my own personal "bluebook." Ironically, I now teach in an evening/weekend program like my father. Excitement about learning and my positive early experiences of the classroom have stayed with me.

But I realized soon after accepting a full-time academic nurse educator position 3 years ago, that my clinically focused graduate program had not been adequate preparation for this role. So, last fall I enrolled in an online graduate certificate in nursing education program, and it's been a great fit. The education electives have been challenging, but humbling, as I've experienced that "fish out of water" feeling so familiar to students who are new to my specialty of maternity. My plan is to take the certified nurse educator (CNE) exam next year.

I've also come to realize that being a novice with new eyes, and a commitment to alternative education, has provided fertile ground for me to construct a new set of questions specifically related to how students access nursing content. Through this program I hope to gain a deeper understanding of the nuts and bolts of nursing education, and thus be better equipped to contribute to the current conversation calling for transformative change. As a nurse educator, I hope to be able to provide for my current students what I have for my homeschooled daughters: an environment where they can feel ownership over their own education, and experience the joy of learning.

My former first grade homeschooler is now a newly minted BSN graduate, and has successfully passed the NCLEX® exam. She was blessed to have had some wonderful role models in her nursing school instructors. She has fallen in love with oncology nursing and, at the time of this writing, is participating in a residency program at Mayo Clinic in Rochester, MN, as well as working on a Bone Marrow Transplant (BMT) unit. Our close circle of friends and family who began as skeptics turned out to be our greatest cheerleaders.

I've offered this very personal family story as inspiration for other nurses who may want to step away from the mainstream in their personal or professional life. There are many ways to share your nursing knowledge, expertise, talents, and passion. And know that your life experiences have value and can inform your professional practice in profound ways. I'll leave you with this advice:

- Don't let the perfect, be the enemy of the good. Be okay with the unsettling feeling that comes along with a new idea that's not yet tied up in a neat and tidy package.
- Just because no one else in the room is saying or doing it, doesn't mean what's in your head is wrong or doesn't have value.
- Don't be afraid to fail. Be a risk taker. But how you do it is up to you.

A Creative in Healthcare

DEBBIE GREGORY, DNP, RN

"Our health system is broken and nurses are poised to be in a position of leadership and disruption."

As a young girl, I had two ideas about the career I wanted to pursue: nurse and interior designer. At the time, the two paths could not have been more diverse. Because I come from a medical family, the "sensible" choice was nursing, and the caring and compassion of nursing appealed greatly to me. My creative and innovative interests were strong, too, but I believed I had to make a choice and limit my creativity, ideas, and inspiration to my home, do-it-yourself projects. This was logical, and life went on for more than 20 years.

One day, a friend mentioned to me that she was going back to interior design school at a local college. My ears perked up, as I was getting ready to be an empty nester, and would have more time to heed my creative call. So I, too, returned to school to study interior design and pursue a love of space planning. While studying the design process and space programming, I felt like my creative side had been set free. My right brain was electrified and turning backflips. I loved every minute of the design thinking, creating and imagining, the intersection of design and function. How can you create spaces that improve function and processes?

Then it happened—our next assignment was to design a healthcare environment. "Oh, this should be a breeze," I thought. "I'll research what the nurses are saying and design it accordingly." To my surprise, there was limited data from nurses in today's environment. Much of the work about designing healthcare spaces centered on Florence Nightingale's work centuries ago. There was a huge void between the design community and the clinical community. My passions collided and I developed a new calling to bridge this gap between nursing and design.

I contacted my nursing school buddy, Laura Buchanan, and shared my epiphany and the discovery I had made about the lack of nursing input in the design of healthcare environments. Laura was a process improvement expert, and I knew she would be interested in evidence-based design and process improvement design. We began seeking out architectural firms, hospitals, and anyone who would listen to us. We knew nurses needed to be informed about the importance of designing their spaces, and architects needed to include nurses on their design teams. We found nurses around the country who were working in design, and created an organization to bring these minds together. Everyone thought that they were the only ones doing this work. Thus, the Nursing Institute for Healthcare Design (NIHD) was formed. We shared our vision for nurses to be at the design table, educated and equipped to advocate for healthcare design spaces. Many conversations in the design industry were challenged with questions about what the nurse's role might be, or how this knowledge could be impactful to the design of hospitals.

Advocating for the clinical voice at the healthcare design table is the mission of NIHD. The organization has grown to include nurses and members from all areas of healthcare design. Today, a nurse space planning and design clinical track is a cornerstone of the Healthcare Design Conference, and we have published a book, *Nurses as Leaders in Healthcare Design: A Resource for Nurses and Interprofessional Partners*. Partnerships have been formed with architecture and design organizations, industry leaders, manufacturers, universities, and many others to bring the clinical perspective to the design of healthcare spaces. NIHD is dedicated to educating and inspiring nurse leaders to promote the clinical voice in the design of healthcare. Moving forward, it is a dream to expand our mission to include innovation and entrepreneurship as a platform for change and transformation.

This pioneering journey was a great challenge that created the hybrid profession to satisfy both sides of my brain. Evolving this vision to the next level meant getting my doctorate in nursing practice (DNP). Being able to navigate at the executive level for healthcare transformation required more education and training. After receiving my DNP in innovation and leadership, I continue to see that nurses are still having to put their creativity and innovative spirits on the shelf. It is now my passion to empower nurses to bring their creativity forward, combine design thinking in all aspects of healthcare, and be a catalyst to transform healthcare in the United States. Our health system is broken, and nurses are poised to be in a position of leadership and disruption. There are things I will do differently this time—lessons I have learned along the way that I would like to share to help others on this journey.

First, FIND YOUR TRIBE. The work of Margaret Wheatley (2006) rings true in creating new ideas and order among chaos. She says, "Seeing the interplay between system dynamics and individuals is a dance of discovery that requires several iterations between the whole and its parts" (p. 143). When you "see" something that needs a solution but can't quite put your arms around it, it's imperative to find others who are passionate, courageous, and life-giving. Many of those closest to you may be left brain dominant. They will not understand your ideas and will focus on the parts rather than the whole. It's key to surround yourself with right-brained people during this stage. Analysis paralysis, business models, financial pressures, looking through the lens of a microscope—these can kill the creativity and energy needed to look at the entire system and develop solutions. Find your tribe!

Second, TRUST YOUR INSTINCTS. Creative people working in math and science industries, such as healthcare, engineering, and accounting, can find it difficult to find the support and empowerment needed to take steps into the unknown. Many in these more rigid and prescriptive environments cannot move forward without a defined timeline and strategic road map. Often, pioneering paths do NOT have road maps or defined paths. It's the creative entrepreneur who sees the goal at the end, and then finds a way to get there—almost a reverse strategy that keeps the endgame in sight while maneuvering throughout the process to get there. This is a unique leadership skill called *adaptive leadership*, using intuition and improvising. You may have a deep sense of knowing that does not require analysis or evidence. Empathy is a component of adaptive leadership and is a foundational competence in nursing.

Many nurses may possess adaptive leadership skills but have not been empowered to explore them. Trust your instincts!

Third and most important, REJECT FEAR. According to Tom and David Kelley at IDEO, the biggest fears that hold us back are: "the fear of the messy unknown," "fear of being judged," "fear of the first step," and "fear of losing control." In their article, "Reclaim Your Creative Confidence," they discuss pushing past fear and just taking the next step. And, as highlighted in Frank Zilm's article titled *The Creative Mind*, Donald MacKinnon suggests that "courage may be the most important component of creativity" (2018). Being able to follow one's intuition rather than logic and imagine the impossible are keys to innovation. This requires a constant "pep talk." You need to be aligned with a group that is going to cheer, correct, and champion your path with you. Having a tribe to hear and co-create with is a special gift. Reject fear!

Just so you know, I have to constantly "preach" these lessons back to myself daily. It's not the kind of process that provides a definitive conclusion of understanding. You grow along the journey and learn more and more about yourself and what makes you tick. This is where my new passion and mission comes in: a supporting structure for nurses who want to explore creativity and innovation. A welcoming tribe to inspire, explore, empower, and encourage the creative process and to really take a hard look at healthcare and find solutions. This I know: together, with the right tools and vision, we can make a difference.

SUPPLEMENTAL RESOURCES

- Florence Nightingale and hospital design
  https://kingscollections.org/exhibitions/specialcollections/nightingale-and-hospital-design/florence-nightingale-and-hospital-design
- The Nursing Institute for Healthcare Design
  https://www.nursingihd.com
- Healthcare Design Conference
  https://www.hcdexpo.com
- Nurses as Leaders in Healthcare Design: A Resource for Nurses and Interprofessional Partners
  https://nihd.memberclicks.net/nihd-book-news
- Reclaim Your Creative Confidence
  https://hbr.org/2012/12/reclaim-your-creative-confidence
- The Creative Mind
  https://www.healthcaredesignmagazine.com/trends/the-creative-mind/

The Nurse Attorney

SHAWNA BUTLER, DNP, JD, RN, CPHRM

"ARM NURSES WITH THE KNOWLEDGE NECESSARY TO SUCCESSFULLY NAVIGATE THE CHALLENGING HEALTHCARE INDUSTRY AND ITS POSSIBLE ADVERSE PATIENT EVENTS."

I've had moments when I wish there were one simple word or phrase that easily described my job. In our society, we are frequently asked *what do you do for work? Where do you work?* This, however, is not an easy question to answer for all of us. I am a nurse attorney, and when I tell people that, they give me a puzzled look in return, flustered and confused at the subject. At one time, I too was unaware of this possible career path and I am still evolving through it today, while still definitely excited for the future.

However, the title *nurse attorney* is not an appropriate description of my professional role or career path. I went to nursing school out of high school, intending to obtain a master's degree and become an advanced practice nurse. After being a nurse in an outpatient clinic and an acute care nurse at an academic medical center after graduating with a bachelor's degree, I decided there was not one area of nursing that I loved and wanted to specialize in. Instead, I wanted to be an advocate for both patients and nurses. I decided to go to law school and combine two traditionally unrelated careers. Rather than hold these degrees in separate settings, I used the law degree to arm myself with the ability to advocate for patients and ethical health policy.

After working as a nurse throughout law school (boy was that challenging!) and graduating law school, I began making connections in the quality and safety department at the hospital where I worked. I wanted to combine my two fields: nursing and the law. There are many regulatory requirements that hospitals and healthcare facilities must abide by, and a multitude of required external reporting obligations. By correlating legal language and critical analysis of patient safety events with my nursing expertise, I carved out my own niche within nursing. I finally found the next step of my career journey. A positioned leader at my hospital gave me a great opportunity fresh out of law school, while there were many others who may have had more experience than I. This opportunity set the stage for the rest of my career. Building relationships with people I respected were vital to the development of my professional role.

I continued in this role, while also teaching ethical, legal, and health policy issues to nursing students. I continued to work in patient safety and risk management departments, where I guided our hardworking clinicians on how to handle complex patient events. Initially, I focused on providing solid advice to the clinicians who were involved in an adverse event or medical error. Some were engaged in an patient death or outcome. Other clinicians were officially served as a party to a lawsuit or a complaint against their nursing or medical license. Some were just overworked and struggling with the unrelenting and often unrealistic expectations that the healthcare industry puts on all of us.

As I continuously worked with hardworking clinicians, I began to recognize how our healthcare system is failing nurses everywhere in various ways. Those of us in quality and risk departments do our best to support clinicians, but so much of this work is reactive. I longed for the ability to be proactive in these situations. Clinicians often found themselves as defendants in a lawsuit. They worked so hard with a patient and then felt this boulder of failure on their shoulders. Being a party to a lawsuit does not mean one is sloppy or a poor clinician. Rather, it typically results from a complex patient, in a complex healthcare environment. Systems errors are usually what lead to problems or unexpected outcomes; an error is much less likely to be due to one individual's practice. The healthcare system must be revised so that clinicians are more often successful, and legal problems are prevented. Legal work causes suffering for patients, families, and clinicians.

After working with distraught clinicians, I developed a passion for changing the system. Medical errors are traumatic for those closest to the event. Patients and/or their families are the primary victims who suffer the consequences of these events for obvious reasons. However, the involved clinicians may experience trauma as well, and this is much less known and much less discussed. This phenomenon is known as "second victimization". I focused my doctoral studies on second victimization and the need for clinician support programs in our health systems. Just as "criminal proceedings cause psychological harm to the victims involved," this same trauma can occur for clinicians, as well (Ortho, 2002, p .314). "Physicians, nurses, and other clinicians who are connected to these events often feel somehow responsible. Emotional trauma is frequent. Patient safety expert Albert Wu, MD, MPH, has coined a term for such clinicians: 'second victims.' According to Dr. Wu, the burden that health care providers feel after a patient is harmed, manifesting in anxiety, depression, and shame, weighs so heavily on providers that they themselves are wounded by the event" (Clancy, 2012, para 3). Even beyond the second victimization that occurs after adverse events, there is a volume of other contributing stressors affecting our clinicians. There is compassion fatigue, burnout, moral distress, etc. We need to focus more on wellness and prevention, and free healthcare of unrealistic perfectionist expectations.

As a result, I now work with clinicians early on and throughout their careers. I work to educate and inform them about the realities of their roles, the healthcare system, and how we can create and design healthy workplaces. I want to be a support for them and to teach them how to support each other. I'm trying to arm nurses with the knowledge necessary to successfully navigate the challenging healthcare industry and its possible adverse patient events. My law practice is focused on working with clinicians who may find themselves subject to adversarial litigation in the judicial system and beyond.

I continue to make an effort to remember those who have helped me. Hard work, diligence, and paying attention to my gut was necessary for many high-stress positions. In addition to my professional roles as nurse, patient safety/risk specialist, and educator/professor, I have experienced many other professional endeavors. I present oral and poster presentations at my professional organizations and I write a quarterly legal awareness column in the *Journal of Radiology Nursing*. I continuously search for and secure opportunities to further expand my professional development.

TOP THREE PIECES OF ADVICE

First, be careful who you listen to. Some people have good intentions, but their opinion is not useful and may often be harmful. Pay close attention to whom you respect and why you appreciate them. If you know someone who has managed their finances well, listen to them for financial guidance. If you know someone who has strong relationships, listen to them when it comes to healthy communication and relationships. If you know someone who has had great career success, listen to them regarding their success. However, take all of this with a "grain of salt." What may work for one, may not for another. I had an excellent job as a nurse and it was a risk to go to law school, take on more debt, and have an unknown future. However, it was the correct path for me and it shaped my unique career path. When I have a big decision to make, I typically do not tell anyone, and then announce it after the decision has been made. The chatter of overwhelming input often made it difficult to hear my own thoughts. Your truth may make others uncomfortable and that is okay. I now do intensive research on the topic and weigh the risks and benefits on my own, with minimal input from a few trusted sources.

Second, you want to maintain professionalism, but also be true to yourself. I felt guilty when I was working as a staff nurse, as it did not fulfill me. It was my lifelong dream up until that point. When I embarked on my law school journey, many people criticized my leaving nursing. I knew deep down that my plan would work and it would supplement my nursing, rather than substitute it. We need to be true to ourselves and our passions. If I stayed on as a staff nurse (I still do it per diem, but it is in combination with my other work), I would not be satisfied and would always wonder about my other possibilities. You have to honor what your soul tells you to do. I am always a nurse first, but my nursing path is to help other clinicians directly, so that impacts patients indirectly. It just looks different now.

My final piece of advice is to listen more. Too many people seem to talk for the sake of talking. Speak when it's relevant and meaningful and adds value to the moment—listening is a value of a true leader. A subset of being a good listener is accepting and valuing feedback. Try not to get defensive (it is natural to an extent) and try instead to listen, process, and change where appropriate. We can learn so much from constructive and useful feedback.

SUPPLEMENTAL RESOURCES:

- Pratt, B., Paul, A., Hyder, A. A., & Ali, J. (2017). Ethics of health policy and systems research: A Scoping Review of the Literature. Health Policy & Planning, 32(6). 890–910. doi: 10.1093/heapol/czx003

  https://doi.org/10.1093/heapol/czx003

- State Operations Manual Appendix A: Survey Protocol, Regulations and Interpretive Guidelines for Hospitals

  https://www.cms.gov/Regulations-and-Guidance/Guidance/Manuals/downloads/som107ap_a_hospitals.pdf

- Todaro-Franceschi, V. (2019). *Compassion fatigue and burnout in nursing: Enhancing professional quality of life* (3rd ed.). New York, NY: Springer Publishing Company.

- McAllister, M., & Brien, D. L. (2020). *Empowerment strategies for nurses: Developing resiliency in practice* (2nd ed.). New York, NY: Springer Publishing Company.

- *Journal of Radiology Nursing*

  https://www.journals.elsevier.com/journal-of-radiology-nursing

- Butler, S. (2018). Prevention of communication failures in radiology or procedural/interventional settings. *Journal of Radiology Nursing, 37*(3):145–146. doi: 10.1016/j.jradnu.2018.06.001

  http://www.sciencedirect.com/science/article/pii/S1546084318301226

- Butler, S. M. (2019). Cybersecurity: Why should we be concerned? *Journal of Radiology Nursing, 38*(1):13–14. doi: 10.1016/j.jradnu.2018.12.006

  http://www.sciencedirect.com/science/article/pii/S1546084318302220

- Butler, S. M. (2019). Why Opposition to the criminalization of malpractice is important to patient safety. *Journal of Radiology Nursing, 38*(2):78–79. doi: 10.1016/j.jradnu.2019.04.005

  http://www.sciencedirect.com/science/article/pii/S1546084319300641

- Butler, S. (2019). Do all nurses need malpractice insurance? *Journal of Radiology Nursing, 38*(3):148–149. doi: 10.1016/j.jradnu.2019.05.018

  http://www.sciencedirect.com/science/article/pii/S1546084319301142

The Reflection of a Nurse

PAUL E. COYNE, DNP, MBA, MS, RN, APRN, AGPCNP-BC

"No matter what the obstacles,
you not only deserve fulfillment, you can find it. And,
as a nurse, you are uniquely able to help others find it,
too—which is the most remarkable part of it all."

I was standing in front of a mirror waiting to complete my annual physical exam. As a corporate benefit, Goldman Sachs provided employees the option of having a comprehensive examination in midtown Manhattan. We were dressed in comfortable scrubs, wearing fluffy socks, and received a delicious breakfast while we waited for what, to this day, was the most complete physical examination I have ever had. It was a wonderful company perk for a 26-year-old man in the midst of a wonderful career. Yet, standing there in front of the mirror, I saw a man in scrubs staring back at me saying, "This is who you are." I went home that night and called my mom, dad, and grandmother, and told them I was going to be a nurse.

Four years earlier, at the age of 22, a week after I graduated college, I suffered a left thalamic stroke, leaving me with right-sided weakness, memory loss, and aphasia. The stroke was caused by hypertrophic cardiomyopathy, a genetic heart disease I had been living with since birth. While I had always lived with illness, even having an implantable cardioverter-defibrillator (ICD) implanted since age 15, there is nothing that compares to the struggle of an illness that affects the mind.

During my senior year of college, I received a job offer to work in interest rate derivatives at Goldman Sachs. One month after the stroke, despite not having fully recovered, I was scheduled to begin my career on Wall Street. My family and I felt it was best if I gave it a try, rather than succumb to a life of disability.

I left my loving mom, dad, and grandmother in Massachusetts and moved to Hoboken, New Jersey in this mental and physical state to live with a great friend from college, Vin Cocito, whose support during those years was one of the greatest gifts I have ever received.

Every morning, I would call my parents and they would need to remind me of many things. "Your name is Paul. You work on the 16th floor of 85 Broad Street in New York City. We love you." I didn't tell many people at Goldman Sachs about my medical history. I would use every ounce of energy to overcome my limp when I arrived at work and do my best to fool my colleagues into believing I was operating at 100%. Miraculously, I did well enough to keep my job during the Great Recession without speaking very much. For those first years, most new people I met just thought I was shy.

I went to physical, occupational, and speech therapy for months and spent countless hours on my own, relearning a wide variety of tasks, vocabulary, and previous memories. I kept that job for over 3 years and was fortunate enough to recover to a point where, when I looked in that mirror that day and saw myself in scrubs, I knew who I could potentially be. But I did not believe that it was what I was capable of becoming. A stroke is not kind to the belief in one's intellect.

That negative belief was strengthened within the next year, when my stroke lesion manifested in a new way, and I suffered the first of a series of what was later diagnosed as tonic-clonic spasms. Periodically, my entire right side became extremely rigid, and then convulsed, repeatedly. These episodes took a week or so to recover from fully, as they were physically and mentally jarring. Because of these events recurring at work, I was placed on long-term disability from the role I had worked so hard to maintain.

I faced yet again the same choice that was placed in front of me 4 years earlier: to try or to succumb to a life of disability.

From my personal experience, I knew that the nurse is the role that is best able to heal all aspects of the patient: physical and emotional. I kept thinking about the day when I looked in the mirror and knew who I was supposed to be—someone who would be able to use personal hardship as a force for good and help others even less fortunate.

I did some research on nursing leaders and observed that those who were most able to have broad impact had a doctorate in nursing as well as some form of graduate degree in business, such as an MBA.

While I did not think I was capable enough to achieve this goal, I could not bear the thought of not trying. So, each night, I would write on pieces of paper, "Dr. Paul Coyne" or "Paul E. Coyne, DNP, MBA, MSF, APRN, RN, AGPCNP-BC." I would write it over and over again, night after night, hoping that if I kept writing it, I would believe it was a potential reality. I took the prerequisite courses online and decided that if I was going to go to school, I was going to go all in. I studied for the Graduate Record Examination (GRE) and realized much of my adolescent learning was still fuzzy from the stroke. I relearned my multiplication tables, strengthened my problem-solving skills, and expanded my vocabulary yet again.

I applied to Northeastern University's combined MBA in healthcare management and MS in finance program and Columbia University's combined BSN, MSN, DNP program. I simultaneously attended both schools, and in disbelief of my own capabilities every time I received a new diploma—I completed all five degrees in 4 years.

I didn't believe in my intellect fully until those 4 years were over. The whole time I kept looking for signs that I was on the verge of shaking again or reasons to believe I was still not mentally capable. In that regard, it is still as if I went to sleep crying one night not believing I could become what I dreamed of becoming, and woke up as I walked across the stage with someone handing me a diploma and calling me Dr. Paul Coyne.

Along the way, I passed the NCLEX® exam and became a registered nurse, passed the boards to become a nurse practitioner, completed a subspecialty in palliative care, became published in peer-reviewed journals, and was hired to work as a manager of analytics at New York Presbyterian Hospital, where I studied informatics and analytics.

So, there I was, 30 years old with six degrees, 4 years of work experience at Goldman Sachs, 2 years of analytics experience at New York Presbyterian Hospital, and a clinical expert as a doctorally prepared nurse practitioner. There was finally overwhelming evidence in my mind that I had recovered adequately from the stroke. In addition, I was in a wonderful relationship with a beautiful nurse practitioner named Danialle, whom I met in nursing school. Outside of continuing to live with a heart disease, my life could not have been more set up to have a smooth sail.

In fact, people used to, and still do, tell me, "You did it! Now you can rest and just enjoy your life. Relax." But I was not satisfied to go to work and watch TV the rest of the time. There is nothing wrong with it, it's just not who I am. While I was proud of myself for what I had achieved and very content with my life, I was not optimally fulfilled. Then, I got a phone call from a good friend from nursing school named Mike Wang. He was my study partner at Columbia, and while we would occasionally text, we hadn't seen each other for a couple of years. He called me up and said, "I have an idea that I want to talk through with you. Can you meet me in Starbucks by the nursing school?"

That decision to meet my friend that day changed my life. From that day on, Mike and I have not missed a day of speaking to each other at length. As a result of the business partnership forged that day in Starbucks, and more importantly through the consistent cultivating of a lifelong friendship, I am fulfilled in ways that I never knew were possible.

With my good friend Vin leading the operational aspects of the company, and the addition of a host of new colleagues along the way, we have invented additional products, filed patents, wrote books, published articles, and led research. We have given speeches, served on panels, and had the opportunity to assist other nurses who wish to innovate. We learned how to lead hardware development, software development, mobile application design, marketing, branding, and the creation of artificial intelligence and machine learning healthcare infrastructure. We raised substantial funding, created a corporation, and now serve on its board. We have been recognized by Fast Company, SXSW, Edison Awards, and the American Nurses Association for our creation of iN, the world's first cognitive patient care assistant. Mike and I serve as CEO and president, respectively, of a company that we created: Inspiren.

I remember thinking to myself when Mike asked me to start a company with him, that if I said yes, I would never rest again. But after being part of this remarkable journey, the new question I ask myself is, why would I want to stop? There is so much to do and only one life to do it. After all of this, I have learned that overcoming a stroke, or getting degrees, or achieving professional accolades does not make me successful. Living my life to the fullest makes me successful. What a gift it is to have each day as a chance to achieve a new level of personal fulfillment.

I am most fortunate and grateful for the wonderful family and friends who did not let me settle for anything less than the best version of myself at any point in my life. For the years during my stroke recovery, that motivation was all I had. Now healthy, I still find it hard on some days to stay motivated for this goal. I am, after all, a human being. But on those days, they lift me up. Danialle is now my wife and pregnant with our first child. I can honestly say I am fulfilled.

I decided to share my personal story in this book to add my voice to the chorus of even more inspirational nurses. I hope those reading this will further realize that the sky is truly the limit for the nursing profession, and for each and every nurse. No matter what the obstacles, you not only deserve fulfillment, you can find it. And, as a nurse, you are uniquely able to help others find it, too—which is the most remarkable part of it all.

- Decide who you want to be; then envision it, believe it, and become more than you dreamed.
- No matter how hard you doubt, try anyway.
- Achieving success and fulfillment does not have an end. It is a lifelong pursuit.
- The right people must be in your life who desire for you to be the best version of yourself.

SUPPLEMENTAL RESOURCES

- Northeastern University, School of Nursing
  https://bouve.northeastern.edu/nursing
- Columbia University, School of Nursing
  http://www.nursing.columbia.edu

- Wittmann-Price, R. A., Thompson, B. R., & Cornelius, F. H. (2017). *NCLEX-RN® EXCEL: Test success through unfolding case study review* (2nd ed.). New York, NY: Springer Publishing Company.
  https://www.springerpub.com/nclex-rnr-excel-second-edition-9780826128331.html
- New York Presbyterian Hospital
  nyp.org
- Fast Company
  https://www.fastcompany.com
- SXSW
  https://www.sxsw.com/conference/health-and-medtech
- Edison Awards
  https://www.edisonawards.com
- the American Nurses Association
  https://www.nursingworld.org
- Inspiren
  https://inspiren.com

The Rebel Nurse's Progress Note

A highlight of being innovative is taking your unique passion and applying it to something new, ultimately creating an explosive change for the better. These rebel nurses, just like yourself, dared to think outside the box and allowed their nursing skill set to cross barriers. Whether you're a millennial nurse perfectly situated to keep up in the fast-paced environment of changing healthcare, or a nurse willing to take a risk, whatever you do, be willing to advocate for the vulnerable and voiceless. And know that even in the places of doubt, decide what you want to be and then envision it. In this way, you'll find that there are successful methods of failure that will push you to find your confidence and help you grow.

Although sometimes life will just *happen*, be open to the change, respond to your gut, and work hard. As nurses, we can do many things, but having a willingness to jump into unfamiliar waters will give you the unique opportunity to re-define what it means to be a "nurse" in today's society. With time, like these nurses, you'll start developing leadership skills that allow you to create influence and create more opportunities for decision-making. As long as you're willing to be bold and embrace your value, you are sure to prevail across many sectors.

What sphere are you interested in embracing that may seem outside the norm of your typical profession or everyday routine? How could you use a unique skill set or passion you have been pushing aside to ultimately influence how problems are solved in nursing?

4

The Price of Compassion: Soulful Stories of the Humanity of Nursing

Nursing is not just evaluating patient symptoms, dressing wounds, lab work, and value-based care—nursing impacts the soul in each of us. In our weakest places, in our most vulnerable areas of life, nursing has literally opened the door to the most painful, but most rewarding moments in the lives of others. The dying, the hurt, the raw, emotional places of life: nurses have the privilege to walk in these spaces and provide a comforting hand, a compassionate touch, and a life-changing presence. Journey with these nurses as they share the deeply intimate and amazing moments in their lives and the lives of those they care for. Enter the space of nursing that has paid the price of compassion.

The Gift of Nursing

ELIZABETH TONER, MJ, MSN, RN

> "WE MUST NEVER LOSE SIGHT OF THE MOMENTS WHEN WE
> CLEARLY SEE THE ACTIONS WE, AS NURSES, CAN TAKE."

Sunday, February 15, 1981—the first day of the last week of my father's life.

"*He's dying*," I mull over the words in my head, "*he should be dead already. We've said good-bye to him already.*" While I don't say any of this, it's true. At least twice in the last 6 weeks of my father's final decline, my mother, 12-year-old sister, and I have stood at his bedside to say goodbye. Each time, he has rallied after a fashion; a thin shadow of his former self, never quite well enough to come home, simply temporarily pulled back from the brink. While he is, in fact, dying, he has no active infection, no symptoms that require skilled medical treatment. So, they are discharging him.

Thirty-eight years later, I struggle to analyze the events of that day—that week—with the eye of an RN, but they lack the continuity necessary for me to make any real conclusions.

One crystal clear memory of that day is of my father at home for the first time in 6 weeks, since a brain tumor (metastases from his lungs and liver) claimed his cognitive processes. Before he left, he had, at turns, claimed his bowl of chili was filled with maggots and taken all the cushions off the sofa and stuffed them into the cupboard behind the bar. His coup de grace was his attempt to move a heavy wooden love seat up the steep back stairway at 5 a.m. When he'd gone into the hospital, he'd been thin, bald, with an ill-fitting wig that hung strangely around his ears.

Now he is gray-skinned, skeletal, his blue jeans hanging off his bony frame and his shoulder blades prominent through the blue knit of his polo shirt. Daddy is sitting on the stairway landing, his expression childlike and his chest heaving with the effort of getting from the car, through the entryway, and up three or four steps toward the first floor. He is 5'11", but he looks so small and diminished. I want to say something, to comfort him. But nothing in my 14 years has given me the language, the words to give him back his dignity—this man who used to bound up this staircase two steps at a time. So I remain silent, standing on the stairs beside him, looking down at him, as if I'm a spotter for a gymnast.

My next memory: Daddy, now in his plaid pajamas, propped up on a pillow on his side of the bed. There is a copy of the *Milwaukee Sentinel* folded in half next to him on the 1970s green quilted bedspread, and a Cross pen and a yellow legal pad on the nightstand. He is trying to read and write, but the feeble scratches on the paper tell me that even his favorite tasks elude him. I will find those plaid pajamas, empty, on the front seat of the station wagon, just 5 days later, folded neatly as if waiting for him to return from the airport.

I feared and hated hospitals for a long time after that. I avoided people who were dying. I avoided friends with family members who were dying. Then, a serendipitous turn of events landed me in nursing school 28 years later. On a similar February day of 2009 in a Pennsylvania hospital room, I confronted the demons of that Wisconsin winter.

I am 42 and a second-semester community college nursing student, which is to say I have almost no helpful clinical skills, although I've gotten reasonably good at giving bed baths without having to run out of a patient's room 20 times for supplies. It is a Saturday clinical day and my assigned patient is decidedly low-maintenance, her needs cared for quickly. So I begin patrolling the hallway on our unit, looking for classmates who might need help.

As I pass the room of a patient I had cared for the previous week, Laurie—one of my favorite nurses—bursts out of it, looking frazzled and a bit frantic. "Can I help you?" I ask, expecting she'll say no, figuring it's something out of my scope of practice, but to my surprise, she says, "Actually, yes, since you know him. He's had fecal emesis and really needs cleaning up, but I want to call his doctor and get him on hospice and get him a morphine drip." Even as a nursing student, I feel the weight of her words, for the patient, for his family, and for Laurie. Fecal emesis means he is vomiting stool—a sure sign that his cancer (which I know began in his liver) has created a blockage somewhere in his intestines. The morphine drip will control his pain and ease, but also slow his labored breathing. This man is nearing the end of his life. I take a deep breath and nod, feeling deeply uncertain. Laurie murmurs a breathless "thanks" and rushes off to make her phone calls.

Before entering his room, I stand for a long moment in front of the supply shelves, determined to get everything I think I might need. Wash basin. Emesis basin (just in case). Soap. Two spare gowns. Lots of towels. Plenty of washcloths. Oh, and mouthwash. I unceremoniously dump everything but the towels into the basin, then pile them on top, wondering yet again why the hospital is the place where you are subjected to the roughest, scratchiest towels. Seems to me if you're dying, you deserve to be dried off with towels from the Plaza Hotel.

Back in the hallway, I take another deep breath and knock lightly, then push the door open and close it quickly behind me. The patient glances up, but I sense he isn't really seeing me. His eyes are distant, his skin dusky. I smile with what I hope looks like compassion and sympathy. "Let's get you cleaned up, OK? I'm sure you're not feeling great." He nods, as if to say, "Nursing students—always stating the obvious."

I tug multiple pairs of latex gloves out of the box on the wall, and lay them on his bedside table. Twisting the faucet at the wash sink, I let the water run until it's luxuriously warm, then squirt the green liquid that passes for hospital bodywash into the basin and fill it with water, watching the bubbles form. As I set the brimming bucket on the table and don a pair of gloves, I survey the situation. His blue-and-white hospital gown is polka-dotted with brown goo that is beginning to seep into the material, the stains slowly spreading outward. Instead of being repulsed, I find myself filled with determination to do something, *anything* to offer dignity and comfort.

I follow the bed bath routine drilled into our heads the previous semester by a cantankerous and startlingly inflexible simulation lab instructor. I thank her silently now as I remember to uncover one body part at a time, although I prioritize getting the soiled gown off as quickly as I can. It is a slow process because he can do almost nothing for himself, but I don't feel rushed. I say very little—it feels disingenuous to talk about the weather as I would with another patient—but I tell him what I'm doing as I do it. As I wash his abdomen, distended by ascites, my heart aches at the numerous bruises from multiple Lovenox injections.

By the time I finish up, gather up dirty linens, and tidy the room, Laurie enters, pushing the morphine pump, a sign her request for a hospice order has been fulfilled. She nods her approval of my efforts, and, ever the mentor, explains everything she is doing as she hooks up the pump and sets the drip rate. Together, we boost him to a sitting position and get him comfortable. Just in time for his daughter to arrive carrying a cold beer that her father has requested. After greeting her, we quietly exit. My last glimpse of this patient is of him, smiling, seeming much more lucid and chatting with his daughter.

After postclinical conference, I swing by the nurses' break room to thank Laurie. I find her charting through her tears, peering at the computer screen. She turns to me with a tremulous smile and reddened eyes. All she can say is, "If you ever find yourself in a place where this type of thing doesn't make you cry, get out of nursing." I nod and exit quickly, allowing her privacy.

I manage to remain stoic through a three-floor elevator ride and a walk across the parking lot, and even as I pull out onto the street toward home. It is when I roll down my windows to allow the uncharacteristically warm February breeze to blow through my car that the dam finally bursts. Tears begin rolling down my face: tears for my patient, for his daughter, for Laurie; but also for me, for my father, for what we could not have together. Mingled with the grief are tears of joy—joy for the gift nursing has given me: the gift of being able to *do something*, to take action, in the face of the unthinkable, yet inevitable, moments at life's end.

We must never lose sight of the moments when we clearly see the actions we, as nurses, can take. It doesn't have to be at the bedside, but it is essential for nurses to connect to the whole of humanity, to the unique context of every human being's life, even if we do it one person at a time. It is this connection that allows us to change our world—and heal ourselves.

SUPPLEMENTAL RESOURCES

- Matzo, M., & Sherman, D. W. (2019). *Palliative care nursing: Quality care to the end of life*, (5th ed.). New York, NY: Springer Publishing Company.

- Rowles, G. D., & Teaster, P. B. (2016). *Long-term care in an aging society: Theory and practice.* New York, NY: Springer Publishing Company.

- Stillion, J., & Attig, T. (2015). *Death, dying, and bereavement: Contemporary perspectives, institutions, and practices.* New York, NY: Springer Publishing Company.

Walking on the Edge

NANCY HANRAHAN, PHD, RN, FAAN

"Nurses heal the relationship."

At this time in my long career as a nurse, I often consider what was so important about my 45 years as a nurse. What comes after a full career of teaching, practice, and research? What did I learn and why is it important to pass on to the next generation of nurses? Describing what nurses *do* is so difficult, probably because the moments are intimate and precious. Here is a story that left me with a feeling of being on the edge of life and death and making a difference. How do I know I made a difference? The patient and her husband told me, while they cried in each other's arms.

Working as an RN in the ED of a small hospital on the coast of Maine allowed me to be present for the acute care needs of a small community. It was a Sunday in the winter. I started my shift at 7 a.m. Shortly after I arrived, an ambulance alerted us that they were transporting an older woman with metastatic brain cancer for confusion and inability to care for herself. I volunteered to take the case. I met the ambulance at the door and couldn't miss her husband rushing ahead. I directed him to the clerk to get registered. He was highly agitated, screaming that no one ever helped his wife; they only charged him more money.

I looked at his wife on the ambulance stretcher and winced at her look of embarrassment as her husband loudly told everyone that she had had loose bowels all night. The clerk directed him to the admission office, and I reassured him that we would care for his wife while he was gone.

His wife looked scared and didn't take her eyes off me. I got her settled on an exam room stretcher and began my assessment. She appeared in the advanced stages of brain cancer. She seemed to be confused and extremely distressed. I moved slowly, telling her what I was doing with every procedure. She was not able to talk, but it was unclear whether her verbal loss was due to brain cancer or her severe state of distress. I was gentle, and spoke quietly. Eventually, she started to relax. We could hear her husband at the clerk's desk, talking loudly about his frustration and anger that he wasn't getting enough help with his wife, and the cost was unaffordable. I excused myself from his wife, and went to see whether I could help calm him before the scene escalated further.

I directed him to just outside the door of his wife's room. He spoke with loud anger and frustration about the cost of her care and the lack of support. He said, "no one seems to listen to me!" I said I would listen and asked him to tell me everything about what happened during the night. He said she leaked feces all night; as soon as he got her up from the bed and into the bathroom, and cleaned up the sheets and the floor, she would mess again. The whole night was engaged in furiously trying to keep her clean and clean up the feces. I asked him to tell me how he was feeling during this time. He broke into tears and spoke about feeling like a failure and frustrated that the cleanup was endless. He admitted to screaming at his wife to stop but understood that she could not stop defecating. He waited until morning to call the ambulance because he felt he should have been able to handle the situation on his own. He was embarrassed by the condition of the house and the desperate need for help. After a while, he softened his speech and started to cry. He looked exhausted. I gently drew him back into the room to stand by his wife's side.

His wife was weeping, as was he. They made soft, tender exchanges that seemed to acknowledge the suffering they both shared. I began by talking about the previous night as a horrible experience that is not uncommon when people with brain cancer move into later stages of the illness. I said it was a severe alert to their need for sustained help. They both nodded. They looked at each other, with tears in their eyes. Their suffering seemed bottomless, and I knew these types of illnesses could go on endlessly. They needed to connect with their strength.

I turned to her husband and asked him how long they had been together and how they met. He looked gently and lovingly into his wife's eyes and told the story of first seeing her ice skating. She was beautiful, graceful, and strong. They became a couple and married 3 months later. They lived together for 60 years. As this beautiful memory held all of our attention, the suffering eased. They tightly held hands and listened to me as I gave them a synopsis of their next steps. She would be admitted to the hospital, and a better support system could include home care or hospice. Finding comfort would likely be the focus of the next stages of their care. I noted the beauty, grace, and strength of their relationship as a place to return when they needed to find respite from the suffering. They nodded their heads and looked at each other tenderly.

As the stretcher wheeled out of the ED, with the husband in tow, I thought about the transaction. I knew from my experience as a nurse that people may think that no one wants to hear such details. However, it is in the sharing of the suffering that makes it possible to continue to bear the pain. The husband was in an extreme state of stress when he arrived in the ED. He was angry, frustrated, and scared. He yelled out his frustration to the clerk and other staff. It was clear he was concerned about the cost of his wife's healthcare. I intervened. I listened with care, asked questions to help him recall the painful details of his experience. He described being alone and powerless over his wife's cancer. As he spoke, his stress level appeared to decrease; he cried as he acknowledged the deep pain of his helplessness and the loss of his beloved wife. I was aware that his wife was probably experiencing the same helplessness and grief, but also feeling ashamed that her condition was so out of control and negatively affecting her husband.

Nursing care in the ED is usually a brief intervention because of the demand for quickly triaging patients to hospital beds or home. I was amazed at how effective it was to shift the couple's conversation to a more favorable time. The shift gave them relief from the burden of their current suffering, and introduced the strength that had sustained them for so many years. As they left the ED, I gratefully realized how fortunate I was to be with them at such a critical transition, and to apply my years of nursing experience to achieve greater comfort. I knew they would get excellent care by the nurses in the hospital who would understand that the priority was to address the need for more support for this couple. I believe the couple realized how comforting their relationship could be, even during the worst hours. Sometimes, we all need that experienced person to be present to open doors we cannot open because of our suffering. I will always remember the gift they gave me as they chose to open the door to their foundation of love. I am truly privileged to be invited into such profound moments. Nurses heal the relationship.

SUPPLEMENTAL RESOURCES

- Coleman, D. (1995). *Emotional intelligence.* New York, NY: Bantam.

The Good Nurse

JANIE HARVEY GARNER, RN

> *"We, as nurses, are bound by our passion for nursing*
> *and doing what is best for our patients."*

The day I created the *Show Me Your Stethoscope* community was a day like most others. I went to work at the Veterans Affairs (VA), then went home to make dinner and help my son with his homework. But on that day in September 2015, there was a fire burning in my heart: I heard the women of *The View* lambasting Miss Colorado, a fellow nurse, on national television. How could she think she might win a beauty contest by presenting a monologue about a patient who changed her life, they asked out loud, mockingly. And why was she wearing scrubs as a "costume" and a "doctor's" stethoscope?

I was appalled! A group of powerful women had actively abused and ridiculed a woman in a female-dominated profession on television. What on earth did this fellow nurse—or any nurse, for that matter—do to deserve such criticism? This is when *Show Me Your Stethoscope* struck root.

I was born on Long Island in 1971 to a first-generation Italian immigrant mother and an alcoholic Irish father. I suffered an abusive childhood, with many nights spent protecting my twin sister from my father, throwing myself in between them when his substance abuse led to domestic violence. As I grew up, I decided I would get out of the house and attend college. My grades were pretty decent, and so was my SAT score, and I wanted to put that to good use—to further my education beyond high school. I wanted to be a pediatrician, and more specifically, I wanted to protect children who were vulnerable and suffering at the hands of mentally ill, substance-addicted parents.

I came to learn tuition wasn't cheap and since my parents never considered saving for their children's college tuition a priority, I knew I would have to take out student loans. My father refused to give me copies of his tax returns to fill out a Free Application for Federal Student Aid (FAFSA), and suggested I consider marriage if I wanted to be taken care of. Believe it or not, this conversation took place in 1989—I thought we'd come further than that!

With college out of the question, I opted for Plan B: I enlisted in the U.S. Navy as a hospital corpsman and wound up with a ton of great stories and wild adventures that I will never forget. I figured the GI Bill would pay for my undergrad degree and I could become a Navy officer and a physician that way. While in the Navy, I met a Radioman Second Class and "fell in love." I place that in quotes because, frankly, there was no love involved. I was an abused child still trying to please her father, or in this case my new husband. We had our son Alex in 1993 and divorced in 1995, after a tumultuous and abusive relationship that ended the day he laid his hands upon my son in anger.

I spent the next 7 years barely surviving as a low-income housing project manager, and later as the executive director of a children's charity that operated after-school programs for low-income housing projects. I also managed a McDonald's at night, leaving my son with my mother.

My hard work resulted in the charity winning the Magnolia Award for affordable housing programs. Despite that, I was fired in a fit of temper by the wife of the wife and husband team who ran the charity. Her husband found out about the unfair leasing practices she forced us to follow, and someone had to be blamed and take the fall. And so, I found myself unemployed through no fault of my own, with a 7-year-old son who needed me to provide for him.

Around that time, I met my husband, Paul. We began dating and eventually moved to St. Louis, where he and his family lived. We bought a house and then we had another son. He and I decided it was time for me to put that GI Bill to good use. I had come to realize that all the things I had pictured doing as a physician, were handled and executed by nurses. I knew within my bones and wholeheartedly, I was meant to be a nurse.

And that's when we discovered the GI Bill was only valid within 10 years of my discharge. My college funding was out the window! I'll admit it irked me at first. After all, I had faithfully served my country during Desert Storm and Desert Shield—was it asking too much to have my education expenses covered? But I obtained a job with a local hospital system that provided tuition reimbursement and things started looking okay again.

A friend suggested that I apply to nursing school, but I was a little hesitant. I wasn't sure I was smart enough for college. She dragged me to the entrance exam anyway, and thus began my new schedule of working three or four 12-hour shifts each week while caring for an infant and carrying a full load of classes at St. Louis Community College. The next few years afforded us almost no free time and were full of highs and lows. In the end, though, it all worked out. We couldn't afford daycare during the first year or so, and I only faintly recall my son Ian's second year, but I graduated at the top of my class and, soon after, went to work in a surgical ICU, and then the ED. We bought a house in the country and got the kids into a beautiful school district. Although we were still financially unstable, we were happy.

On February 18, 2011, my world ended. My son Alexander was killed by a distracted tow truck driver. His right leg was amputated and his aorta was torn. He had an unsurvivable head injury. He died before I reached the hospital. Every ED nurse's nightmare had come true for me.

I began working from home facilitating admissions and transfers overnight. Though SSM Health and I disagree on certain things, I will always be grateful that they gave me a chance to work as a nurse when I was unable to leave my house, and when diagnoses such as "complicated grief," "post-traumatic stress disorder (PTSD)," and "panic disorder with agoraphobia" were being thrown around.

In December 2011, I decided I could no longer live without my baby. I drove to a nearby Walmart with three 10-mL syringes full of NovoLog. I spent hours attempting to write my suicide note. And then I thought how ashamed Alex would be if I carried through with it. I decided I needed to do more and I needed to do something GOOD. So, I squirted the insulin onto the pavement, went home, and applied for a job in a local ED.

And that brings us back to September 15, 2015, when I saw a news story about Miss Colorado and *The View*. She had been painted in a terrible light by the show's hosts and I was furious at how those powerful women chose to use their platform to slander a "lesser" woman in scrubs. I decided to create a Facebook group called *Show Me Your Stethoscope* in protest. I thought it apt, as Missouri is known as the "show me state." I expected maybe 30 people from the ED to post pictures of themselves with their stethoscopes, so you can imagine my surprise when 7 days later there were 815,000 healthcare professionals in my group.

These folks told terrific stories about their careers and the patients who changed their lives. I asked myself what I was going to do with this platform (I had started to receive several purchase offers). I decided what I was going to do was GOOD: we would create a voice for nurses throughout the world. I realized the opportunity I had to make Alex proud, to advocate change, and to empower and inspire nurses, moms, families, 815,000 reliable healthcare workers—primarily nurses who wear stethoscopes. And to help with that effort, I formed a team that is still together today.

We, as nurses, are bound by our passion for nursing and doing what is best for our patients. We have tackled issues hospitals would prefer to remain out of the public's view, such as nurse assault and safe staffing. On our mission trips, we have fed an orphanage in Bangladesh and purchased nebulizers for the community around Dhaka. We brought female sanitation supplies to Ghana. We were the first to show up to recent national disasters where we have fed thousands, moved supplies to hundreds of thousands, and supported even more. We have stood by nurses through litigation, assault, violence, and rape. We have made a national stand on safe staffing. We strive to destroy the stigma surrounding substance abuse. We have been invited to work with Facebook and Johnson & Johnson to help bring our efforts to the forefront in healthcare, by taking the path that no other medical professional group has tackled. I am proud to say we have done so with such vigor and zest.

We advocate for nurses every day, as we enter new chapters and challenges as a professional organization. The impossible is what we accomplish every day, and together we are a nation of nurses.

So never lose an opportunity of urging a practical beginning, however small, for it is wonderful how often in such matters the mustard-seed germinates and roots itself.

— *Florence Nightingale*

SUPPLEMENTAL RESOURCES

- 10 Life Lessons We All Need to Learn to Be Successful in Life
  https://everydaypower.com/life-lessons-we-need-to-learn-to-be-succesful

- *Show Me Your Stethoscope*
  http://smysofficial.com
  https://www.facebook.com/showmeyourstethoscopepage
- Campbell, J. C., & Messing, J. T. (Eds). (2017). *Assessing dangerousness: Domestic violence offenders and child abusers*. (3rd ed.). New York, NY: Springer Publishing Company.

The Nurse Iconoclast

KEITH CARLSON, BSN, RN, NC-BC

> *"I'LL ALWAYS BE A CAREGIVER. I'LL ALWAYS BE A NURSE. I'LL ALWAYS BE AN ARTIST. BUT I ALSO KNOW I HAVE TO TAKE CARE OF MYSELF."*

I was born a caregiver. Growing up in a home that looked good on the outside, but wasn't actually happy or functional, I tried hard to please. We weren't allowed to get dirty, and we had to do everything in our power to please our mother. As children, many of our innate impulses were squelched, and that in itself was a form of caregiving, which we observed from our mother that we were reluctant to take part in.

When I was 11, my role as my mother's caregiver changed when my parents divorced on the heels of an affair that led my mother to the man who would become my stepfather—and the love of her life. She moved out of our family home with me in tow and it was just the two of us living on one side of a run-down two-family rental. We were alone together, especially when my soon-to-be step-dad ran back to his wife out of guilt on several occasions.

I learned that love was often associated with being needed, and that giving and caring could—and did—define me.

A TUMOR AND A RAZOR

Jump to 1981, 5 years later. I was 17 years old, and I was visiting my grandparents in their cluttered North Jersey apartment. It was filled with *tchotchkes*, and smelled like underarms, chicken liver, and Juicy Fruit gum.

His face was sallow and gaunt, and his eyes sunken. His neck was loose like a chicken's. But what I really saw looming large in my field of vision was the black tumor on the right side of his face. He was my grandfather, and he was slowly dying. He asked for a shave, and I was hesitant because the tumor smelled a little like rotten meat. Thinking about it, I realized that it probably was indeed rotten meat. I choked back my disgust and prepared his shaving kit.

The shaving cream was the consistency of whipped cream and smelled like vanilla and musk; I smeared it on his face and neck. Gripping the old-fashioned metallic razor in my hand, I slowly worked through his thick beard, revealing the pale yellow skin beneath. I skirted the tumor, leaving a small forest of black stubble around it. He rubbed his smooth face with pleasure as I cleaned up, and I realize now that this likely was his final shave.

REJECTING ART AND EMBRACING CAREGIVING

Because I loved art and had several famous artists on my mom's side of the family, I attended two Philadelphia art schools. I summarily dropped out of both because creating art felt isolating and I couldn't be gentle with my own self-criticism. I wanted to care for others; I wanted to feel connected. Art therapy was very new at the time and I couldn't wrap my head around this unknown field. So I actively subjugated my creativity, a loss that would be felt for decades to come.

In the coming years, I found a calling caring for elders and people with disabilities, and I learned the basics of personal hygiene, medication administration, transfers, and psychosocial care. Becoming a certified yoga instructor and massage therapist, my ability to reach and touch others and soothe their pain was increased exponentially. Massage, yoga, and caregiving were fine, but as a young father of a preteen boy, I needed a well-paying professional career. With several nurses on my dad's side, an obvious realization led me to nursing school and, subsequently, a successful career focused on community health, public health, home care, and hospice.

SOUL DROUGHT

My nursing career continued uninterrupted, until I was a nurse case manager for a very large number of chronically ill, poor patients in the inner city. I was always trying to please, cleaning up the messes in my patients' lives, setting myself up to be a fixer—this almost impossible task broke me as I tried to fix everyone else.

Sharon was a middle-aged Jewish woman with a debilitating disease. Physically frail but powerfully manipulative, Sharon was not similar to my mother on the surface, but nonetheless I was now the caretaker of another exacting Jewish woman who needed more from me than I could give.

Sitting in Sharon's greasy kitchen over cups of herbal tea, I'd fill her pill boxes as she recounted her tales of woe. I bent over backward to help Sharon get control of a life that was always out of control, but Sharon was only one of the many patients I was attempting to fix.

That powerful need to fix everyone, to be everything to everyone, created an insidious slide into burnout. And what's a conscientious, capable, and caring nurse to do when he's burning out? He works harder. He works more. He presses his nose to the proverbial nursing grindstone and continues on his path "for the good of the patients." If you asked what burnout looked like for me, I'd tell you one thing: it wasn't pretty.

Burnout was like ropes of obligation knotted in my gut. There was this patient to care for, this care plan to write, this crisis to fix. Those ropes knotted together more and more tightly, like the rubber bands on the wind-up planes we'd fly around the yard as kids. Burnout was like a ball and chain dragging along with every step.

In the midst of this, my stepfather developed pancreatic cancer. My wife and I moved in with him and my mother, taking turns sleeping on the couch for the last 3 weeks of his life. After all, I was the only nurse he trusted. We were there with almost my entire immediate family when he took his last breath. Once again, I was set up to care for my mother, but this time in widowhood.

The pain of my numerous obligations lodged in my body, and my mind reeled with despair. Those walks with my wife? They didn't happen. My creative impulses? Gone. My ability to socialize normally? Out the door. My psyche was filled with the needs of my patients like an overinflated tire ready to burst. As a burned-out nurse, my compassion was worn thin.

It wasn't just compassion fatigue—I was compassion-starved. Or as my dear friend, the wise nurse author Carol Gino, once said: "*It's not compassion fatigue, it's 'soul drought.'*" My ability to be fully present with my patients was lost. My center was gone and my compassion was blunted. The drought was deepening. Was I still the caregiver I was born to be? Did nursing do this to me? No, it wasn't nursing—I did this. The reservoir was dry and I flew my flag of martyrdom high.

RISING FROM THE DEPTHS

When I recognized that this overwhelming giving and caring had become my false North Star, I was lost. When your compass has no true north, where do you turn? I credit my wife, Mary, with saving me.

First, like in a 12-step program, I—a burned-out nurse addicted to caregiving—had to admit that I had a problem. My recovery involved a leap of faith, a change of gears, quitting that damn job, and finding work where less direct care was required.

I learned to live again, to embrace a life that didn't solely revolve around caring for others. It was a life that embraced a balance between life and work, where creative pursuits were a root of my joy, and where caring for patients was not the central focus of my existence.

That little boy afraid to get dirty for fear of mom's reaction is still inside me. That teenager who gave my grandfather his final shave still has a voice. And that nurse who twisted himself into knots is just beneath the surface.

I'll always be a caregiver. I'll always be a nurse. I'll always be an artist. But I also know I have to take care of myself. And that flag of martyrdom? I burned it.

THE NURSE ICONOCLAST

I've always done things differently throughout my life. I was an art school dropout while my friends continued the creative slog. I slaved away in restaurants and bars, saving enough to buy a one-way ticket to Europe, departing just after my 21st birthday to hitchhike for 11 months, taking in the art, architecture, and history that fascinated me.

As a massage therapist, I worked with people with AIDS, often on their death beds, lovingly caring for a tight-knit community of gay men slowly succumbing to the disease in the days before antiretrovirals. When no one wanted to touch their Kaposi sarcoma lesions and recommended I use gloves, I rejected that idea and offered skin-to-skin contact for those in such need of compassionate touch. And once I left direct care nursing, my iconoclastic nature again came into focus. I established myself as one of the first nurse bloggers before we knew what it was really all about. I jumped on the podcasting bandwagon and launched one of the first nursing podcasts on the planet. And when coaching came into my field of vision, I was among the first group of nurses to become a board-certified nurse coach (NC-BC), a new designation giving nurse coaches increased credibility as recognized by the American Nurses Association (ANA). Middle age has been about coming into my own and realizing what gifts I have to give. It's been decades of self-inquiry to get me to where I stand today.

As a career coach, I help nurses sort out their career-related issues. Some clients' problems are relatively simple: update the resume, prepare for a job interview, apply to school, and create a LinkedIn profile. But others face much more existential issues: divorce, burnout, bullying, a loss of direction, depression, an empty nest, a crisis of faith in nursing, medicine, and healthcare. They all come to my metaphorical door and I welcome them with open arms.

As a blogger, freelance writer, podcaster, career coach, and motivational keynote speaker, my role as a nurse is vastly different than most, but I'm still a nurse. Do I shave around tumors and dress wounds? Not anymore. Rather, I provide soulful care for nurses in distress that only a nurse can truly give, and I advise on nursing careers and life transitions that a fellow nurse can more readily understand.

Being born a caregiver is a gift, and finding my optimal caregiving role is an even greater one. Nurses need help and this nurse iconoclast does his best to assuage the pain felt by nurses from every walk of life.

SUPPLEMENTAL RESOURCES

- Nurse Keith's Digital Doorway (blog)
  http://digitaldoorway.blogspot.com
- Nurse Keith Website
  http://nursekeith.com
- The Nurse Keith Show (Podcast)
  https://nursekeithshow.libsyn.com
- Speeches
  https://www.youtube.com/watch?v=lud0Kneb4Jg&t=69s
- Board Certified Nurse Coach information
  https://inursecoach.com
- Multibriefs News Service
  http://exclusive.multibriefs.com/author/keith-carlson
- Todaro-Franceschi, V. (2019). *Compassion fatigue and burnout in nursing: Enhancing professional quality of life. Workbook for overcoming nurse stress and burnout.* New York, NY: Springer Publishing Company.

The Mindfulness Nurse

DEBBIE TOOMEY, RN, CIPP

"I TURNED MY STRESS INTO HAPPINESS."

My journey began many years ago when I was working as a bedside nurse. I felt stressed like many of my hard-working colleagues. The pressures and demands pushed many of my nursing colleagues to tread home crying or leave entirely to work for another hospital. Those who worked there as long as I had, only stayed for the perceived "golden handcuffs." Many seasoned nurses felt sentenced to their jobs because of a top-scale salary and seniority benefits.

I have always valued health and happiness, which is the main reason I went into nursing. I wanted to help people feel better, and I experienced that healing power in the beginning of my career in the early 1990s. But as the healthcare system changed, it brought many challenges that healthcare professionals had to face head on, with no warning. During these years, I felt my nursing practice and my values compromised; I was not providing the nursing practice that I was taught to do. I had so little time to talk with my patients and take care of them. The new way of caring for people was working with less and doing more. I became jaded and apathetic. I lost sleep. I gained weight. I felt anxious. Basically, I was neither healthy nor happy; I was tired, physically and emotionally.

While I knew the importance of stress management and preventive ways to live a healthy and happy life, I was tired of taking care of hundreds of patients with stress-related ailments over the course of 30 years. Being a Filipina, I was fortunate to come from a family of doctors, pharmacists, and spiritual healers who embraced both Eastern and Western philosophies of health and healing. To me, combining both models of healthcare was economical and sensible. Each form of medicine relied on the power of the other.

I witnessed the disconnection of the healthcare philosophy in the United States, and I wanted to fill the gap by offering research-proven Eastern and Western wellness techniques that could promote better health and healing. I wanted to educate and empower people on how to take better care of themselves, through easy-to-do techniques that could restore and rejuvenate their whole being. Moreover, I wanted to put the responsibility of self-care and wellness back into the hands of people. It was my dream to establish my own company. I wanted this dream badly, but I did not know how to begin.

Then, something happened one sunny morning that changed my life. I was awakened by a voice that said, *"Do stress management workshops."* It was loud enough to wake me from a deep sleep, and when I looked around in my bedroom to see who said it, there was nobody there. It wasn't my husband because he was downstairs preparing breakfast for our three boys. I turned over to one side, hoping to change the channel of this weird dream. Again, I heard, *"Do stress management workshops."* I rolled over the other way and put one pillow over my ear to try to get more sleep. Again, the Voice said, *"Do stress management workshops."* Before I knew it, I said, "NO! I can't. I don't know how to do workshops!"

I forgot about this incident for the rest of that day, but was reminded of it every morning for the next 2 weeks. Like an alarm, it kept waking me up. Eventually, I changed from dismissing the Voice to challenging and asking it for guidance. I decided to go for it. It was a magical time. I started to understand how Neale Donald Walsch, author of *Conversations with God*, must have felt. I remember listening for instructions and asking for directions. I kept asking for signs, symbols, and synchronicities to prove to myself I was not hallucinating. But the Voice never failed me. It always gave me the answers I needed to move forward in turning the stress management workshops into a reality.

A month later, I taught my first stress management workshop, and continued to offer it for almost 1 year. In my classes, I checked the participants' blood pressures and taught mind-body-spirit practices, such as breathing techniques, the power of positive thinking, aromatherapy, laughter, yoga, and so much more. We all looked forward to our weekly time together. I didn't know it back then, but I was on my way to starting my own company. Because of that experience, I developed a "go for it" and "show-up" mindset that has helped me push through my insecurities.

I turned my stress into happiness. One year later, I started my company Ultimate Healing Journey, LLC. It was a company that offered stress management programs, intuitive readings, and integrative wellness coaching. My job stress lessened as I pursued a new purpose in health and healing. Healthcare institutions and visiting nursing companies hired me to be their wellness speaker when they offered "lunch and learn" marketing programs and corporate retreats. Also, I partnered with a coaching company in California, and did monthly intuitive readings over the phone for its global clients. I did all of this while I worked part-time as a nurse.

I am thrilled to share that I am in the 10-year trajectory of an "overnight success." While overnight successes do occur, they are few and far between. Starting and sustaining a business requires hard work, overcoming fears, and having amazing coaches and mentors. As of this writing, I am still working as a nurse part-time, still living two different lives, but I have branded myself as the mindfulness nurse. My hospital awarded me a nurse fellowship award to do mindfulness training for medical–surgical nurses. I tested this training by doing a pilot study that involved 40 nurses. Doctors and nurses have asked me to speak on self-care, mindfulness, and stress management.

For my company, I have thus far published three books, and am proud to report that Pelham High School in New Hampshire is using my book, *The Happiness Result*, for their course, "Managing the Mind." School officials have told me the students are enjoying the course and applying the techniques to help them in their lives. While I no longer do intuitive readings for people, I teach my clients to listen and trust their inner voice and to take the best actions toward reaching their goals. I have been hired to do keynotes, trained companies on positivity in the workplace, and coached many business leaders. My hospital bought 500 copies of my book, and gave them to nurse leaders and novice nurses after they completed their orientation training. Finally, I have led a self-care and resiliency training retreat that has been well received by many stressed and burned-out healthcare professionals.

The more I speak in front of nurses and other healthcare providers, the more I get asked how I got started. While there are so many pearls of wisdom I learned along the way, here are three to get anyone started in the direction of their dreams.

1. **Know what you want**. The more you know what you want, the quicker you will find it. Imagine that the universe is ready to serve you; all you have to do is let it know what you want. A good place to start is what you believe in. Then imagine what that would look like as a business. Do your research and talk with others who are already doing it.

2. **Know where to draw your line**. Don't ever feel powerless and stuck. Don't allow yourself to be held captive by a "golden handcuff." There is always something you can do to make your life better. To help yourself from feeling stuck, start taking classes to refine your skills. If you want to be a speaker, join clubs like Toastmasters to help yourself be a speaker.

3. **Know who will cheer you on and coach you.** Embarking on a new venture such as starting your own company can be daunting and lonely. It can bring up many fears and insecurities. Be with people who believe in you. Hire coaches who can help you stay accountable to your business goals. Have mentors who can guide you and keep you grounded. You are the sum of all the people you spend time with. Choose wisely.

After 20 years of a myriad of mind-body-spirit training, I feel the "golden handcuffs" slowly melting away. The fearful and empty feelings have been replaced with hope and happiness, as I created and cultivated my own "nurse resilience toolkit." This toolkit has been a game-changer in both my personal and professional life. I now teach these lessons in my self-care and resiliency training courses.

I believe it's time for nurses to stop suffering at work. Nurses need training to help them prevent and manage their stress. Although research consistently shows that workplace stress is increasing for nurses, ongoing training for self-care and stress reduction is not being offered. Chronic job stress is the elephant in the room that is not being addressed fully or taken care of in hospitals and healthcare organizations. Nurses deserve more. They need to be given the time to take care of themselves at work without shame. Self-care and resiliency training is a must for nurses in order for them to thrive in the current work climate. My company is committed to educating and empowering nurses to show them how to create and cultivate their own "nurse resilience toolkit" in person and online.

Here are a few parting words for any nurse or healthcare provider who is suffering from job stress and burnout. Pause. Listen to your body. Pay attention to who or what depletes your energy or refuels your energy. Finally, follow the Voice of your heart. When you do, you will be able to turn your stress into happiness.

SUPPLEMENTAL RESOURCES

- Health and Happiness
  https://healthandhappinessspecialist.com
- Walsch, N. D. (1997). *Conversations with God: An uncommon dialogue.* New York, NY: Putnam.
- Ultimate Healing Journey, LLC workshop
  http://www.ultimatehealingjourney.com
- Toomey, D. L. (2016). *The happiness result: More time, more health, more love, more success.* Quincy, MA: Borromeo Publishing.
- Youtube Channel:
  https://www.youtube.com/channel/UC3s4Mwq9uWudFWdhqJNyroQ
- Todaro-Franceschi, V. (2019) *Compassion fatigue and burnout in nursing: Enhancing professional quality of life. Workbook for overcoming nurse stress and burnout.* New York, NY: Springer Publishing Company.
- McAllister, M., & Brien, D. L. (2020). *Empowerment strategies for nurses: Developing resilience in Practice* (2nd ed.). New York, NY: Springer Publishing Company.

A Search for Meaning

NOAH HENDLER, MSN, MPS, RN, APRN, FNP-C

"I AM COMMITTED TO MAKING SURE MORE NURSES SEE THEMSELVES AS BELONGING AT THE FOREFRONT OF HEALTHCARE INNOVATION."

In my 20s, no one could have convinced me that I would become a nurse. It was not that I thought poorly of the profession; I did not think of it at all. When most of my undergraduate classmates at Duke University were focused on their careers and interviewing with investment banks, law firms, or medical schools, I was focused on interviewing people about their religious beliefs. As a sophomore, I took a class on American religious cults with a professor who lectured about a faith, and thereafter brought people who practiced it to meet the class. Beliefs varied widely, but each person who came to the class had found substantial meaning in their lives. When the course ended, I wanted to find meaning, too.

My search began with writing a proposal and, much to my surprise, being awarded a few grants to begin collecting people's spiritual autobiographies. I would interview them on how their beliefs arose, how they practiced, and how they led their lives. I photographed everyone I interviewed. The work was transformative for me and, in retrospect, key to my personal development, but it also earned me some recognition as a photographer and documentarian. Soon after graduating with a degree in comparative religion, I was awarded a fellowship aimed at placing young documentarians with international nongovernmental organizations. For me, this meant going to Rwanda, a country still emerging from recent war and horrific genocide.

In Rwanda, I photographed children orphaned by war, living alone in homes with no adult support or supervision. This project helped establish, within the United Nations and international donor community, that Rwanda's child-headed households were a new category of vulnerable children in need of their own specific programs and funding. It also led to other opportunities, creating publications advocating for vulnerable populations worldwide, such as victims of landmines in Southeast Asia, internally displaced people in Azerbaijan, villages ravaged by AIDS in Malawi, and immigrants from Mexico to the United States, and from Russia to Israel.

While I developed as a professional photographer, documentarian, and publisher, the Internet was also taking shape. Clients began asking me to help them publish online as well as in print. I enrolled in a graduate program at New York University (NYU) focused on teaching technology to artists and other nontechnical people. I became part of a group of misfit technologists, all crammed into a downtown loft, unknowingly laying the groundwork for what would become New York's Silicon Alley. I learned how to build sensors and software, but most importantly how to think about technology and design. I began to practice what is now called design thinking, iterating through feedback loops of technical and business development, but I definitely was not yet thinking about nursing. Even though I was busy with projects related to healthcare, like publishing a book detailing the role of chaplains in hospitals, or making software for geriatric facilities, I was not at all interested in providing healthcare.

Yet, when one of my best friends became sick with leukemia, I found myself drawn to his bedside. Like the chaplains whom I spent months shadowing had done for their patients, I stayed in his room as others drifted in and out. I finally noticed nurses while sitting at his bedside. From my dying friend's point of view, it was hard to miss them. Nurses were omnipresent. They were the ones who continually cared for him. They often looked beyond his diagnosis and treatments to help him deal with the ramifications of being ill, and ultimately contend with his own mortality.

When my friend died, so did a part of me. I felt adrift, nearly back to where I started on my initial search for meaning as an undergraduate. Nothing seemed to mean much. Making photographs, publications, software—all of it was trivial. I needed to contribute in a more direct way, but did not know how to do so. The most direct contributors I knew were the nurses who touched and tended to my friend. I realized I was more like them than anyone else I knew; I too liked caring for people. This simple fact seems obvious now, but it was a bit of a revelation then. I was raking leaves on an appropriately solemn fall day when the thought occurred to me. I dropped my rake, ran inside, and excitedly told my wife that I was a nurse. She had no clue what I was talking about. After all, I was not actually a nurse. I had never even studied anything health related, nor did I secretly hold a nursing license, but I was most certainly a nurse at heart; I only had to become one literally.

There were frequent taunts from friends, family, and colleagues about wanting to be a nurse. Few understood my decision. They referred to me as "Nurse Focker," after Ben Stiller's character in the film *Meet the Parents*, who, like me, is a rare breed of male, Jewish nurse. Most could not grasp why I wanted to enter the profession. I was determined, and was used to forging my own career path. After completing prerequisite courses, I enrolled in an accelerated bachelor's degree program. Soon enough, I emerged an actual licensed RN.

I went to work in an ED. The job was trial-by-fire, and I loved it. I felt like I was using skills and strengths I developed elsewhere. Quickly building rapport with patients came naturally; I'd spent years quickly ingratiating myself with strangers and photographing them. Even the charged environment of the ED felt oddly familiar, like another kind of war zone. Rapidly assessing, solving problems, making a tangible impact, and being helpful—especially in the midst of a crisis—made the work particularly rewarding.

Creating order from the chaos of traumas, emergencies, and undifferentiated complaints was hard work. By the time I handed a patient off for admission, I felt invested and wanted everything I knew about the person to be passed along. I often watched in disappointment as my patients were handed off to the inpatient team. Much like in the children's game of telephone, essential information about them was lost or distorted.

This communication problem frustrated me enough to try to solve it. I used my expertise in developing software to prototype a process for electronically transferring a patient's hand-off report with greater fidelity. The chief hospitalist dismissed my efforts without even letting me demonstrate my prototype. I was bluntly informed that I was "just a nurse" and should get back to caring for my patients. At the time, I did not know how to respond. I was confused. In my mind, nurses were not "just" anything. I saw myself as a professional who could not only perceive problems, but create solutions. I don't recall even mustering a reply. However, I now see that moment as a formative one. It was when I realized that deploying a full skill set as a nurse would not be easy.

While nurses are trusted more than any other profession, our domain expertise is mistakenly perceived as limited. We are the most pervasive healthcare workforce and in closest proximity to so many healthcare problems. Why are nurses not routinely part of crafting healthcare solutions? I am still asking this question, even after becoming a nurse practitioner, helping start and scale healthcare companies, building products, and leading innovation. Too often I've found myself to be the only nurse in a room filled with people trying to improve healthcare. I am committed to making sure more nurses see themselves as belonging at the forefront of healthcare innovation.

In hindsight, my early career photographing and advocating for others was great preparation for being a nurse innovator. At its core, working with vulnerable people was an exercise in empathy. So, too, was working with technology and beginning to practice design thinking. Empathy is the first step of the design thinking process—one must first relate to people before crafting solutions for them. Empathizing with people, not only caring for them or about them, is essential to making nurses so trustworthy, approachable, valuable, and uniquely positioned to excel as innovators. It is what I admired in the nurses who were with my friend to the end, and why I eventually recognized myself as one of them. I am grateful for realizing this, and remain hopeful that my story, along with so many even more powerful ones in this book, inspires you, too—as a nurse, as an innovator, and beyond.

SUPPLEMENTAL RESOURCES

- Taylor, E. J. (2019). *Fast facts about religion for nurses: Implications for patient care.* New York, NY: Springer Publishing Company.

- Breakey, S., Corless, I. B., Meedzan, N. I., Nicholas, P. K. (2015). *Global health nursing in the 21st century.* New York, NY: Springer Publishing Company.

- Design Thinking for Nurses A free, on line curriculum to help nurses solve complex health and health care challenges

  https://www.nursing.upenn.edu/live/news/1369-design-thinking-for-nurses

- Barry, C. D., Gordon, S. C., & King, B. M. (2015). *Nursing case studies in caring: Across the practice spectrum.* New York, NY: Springer Publishing Company.

The Rebel Nurse's Progress Note

What we imagine you've recognized in your own nursing journey, as well as through the lens of these stories, is that nurses connect to the whole humanity of a person. Nurses, in their essence, heal relationships, use empathy to change distress to peace, and listen, even in the most overwhelming situations. However, as nurses, we should also recognize that sometimes we need help, and that it's necessary and okay to lean on the support of others. As we encourage wellness and prevention in our patients, we must be willing to soulfully take care of our own life's distress. Know where to draw the line for your peace of mind and to be sustainably available for others. Continue to keep up with the spirit of your work—remind yourself of your pride and love of nursing. In an effort to stay balanced:

- As you empathize with others, consider relating to people first, before trying to create solutions.

- Know what you want, both personally and professionally.

- Know who will cheer you on or coach you, because even rebel nurses need support along the way.

> *Where have you felt the sting of burnout or even "soul drought"? Where can you find more balance in your own rebel nurse journey? Where can you transform your own pain into a platform for the greater good?*

Sharing Their Story: Words of Wisdom by Rebel Nurses Who Disrupted the Status Quo

These stories are not meant to make you look down on your own journey, but to motivate you to know that you are the rebel nurse. You are the daring one. The resilient one. Whether you disrupt by accident or by plan, your actions have an impact on the development of healthcare and the patient lives within it. The nurses who have made the strides, the seasoned nurses who have endured the sting, are here to share their story, their wisdom, their moving words to give you the steppingstone for the path of the future of nursing. They are here to help guide you to be the game changer, the trailblazer, and the dedicated, compassionate, and amazing innovator that you are. They are excited to help you embrace that you, too, are the Rebel Nurse!

Lessons Learned

MARTIE MOORE, MAOM, RN, CPHQ

*"Hear what others have to say, learn from their perspectives, but
do not let their mindset limit or dim your passion or vision."*

My senior year final statement from the dean of nursing stated, "Martie will need to find roles that will challenge her mind, or she will be a challenge to manage as a Nurse." Years later, at a dinner for the American Nurses Association Foundation, I learned that Tim Poter-O'Grady, the Foundation's Chair, attended the same college of nursing. Through our shared life experiences, we learned that we were both seen through this same lens by our mutual Dean of Nursing—perpetually questioning, inquisitive minds, refusing to accept this status quo.

Lesson learned: Hear what others have to say, learn from their perspectives, but do not let their mindset limit or dim your passion or vision.

My career track began in the computer science field with data programming and designing data fields. I lived in the Northwest where Microsoft presented data programming as an ever-expanding field of opportunities. Yet, I was deeply dissatisfied. An epiphany dawned on me as I was sitting on a park bench in my hometown. I finally knew I needed to become a nurse. It was uncalled for—there were no nurses at that time in my family. But the need to change course and apply to the nursing program at my local community college was imminent.

I worked as a certified nursing aide, and held two other jobs to support myself and my daughter as I studied the sciences. I had attended college in high school, graduated when I was 16, married my high school sweetheart, and found myself divorced at the age of 19 with a baby girl. This transposition was profound. I struggled to study, work, and complete my clinical rotations. I consistently questioned standard practices such as wound care using Maalox, or not isolating a patient until lab results indicated to do so. These, and other clinical practices, contradicted my instinctive logic. Because of my grades, I was not seen as a student who had the right to question. Yet, I did not let that stop me when I did not agree with the norms within the work setting. I refused to give my chair up to a physician as a student nurse, because I saw us as one team—equals in partnership of healing. I was reprimanded for my refusal.

Lesson learned: Mutual respect influences the culture of safety. Kindness influences the culture of the workplace.

Right out of nursing school, I was hired as the medical coordinator of a neuromuscular clinic for children with developmental disabilities. I had a caseload of several hundred children, and was doing community case management before it was labeled as such. I worked closely with the public health department to advance the health and well-being of the children we mutually cared for throughout both clinical settings. I also served as an expert witness for child protection services. I knew that the system of care for children needed to improve, but felt limited in my knowledge of how to make changes in complex structures such as healthcare.

I returned to school to advance my knowledge and achieve my bachelor's degree in nursing through Saint Martin's University. I worked full-time and studied in the car as my husband drove me to my classes. My daughter did her homework in the backseat. The program that I attended was one of the leading edge programs in adaptation of evidence-based practice (EBP) and the role of nursing beyond acute care. It expanded my knowledge and taught me tools to feed my inquisitive spirit through research and data analytics. Years later, the same university would acknowledge my accomplishments with an honorary doctorate degree in recognition for my service, and accomplishments in advancing healthcare as a nurse leader.

The call to hospital leadership came through an opportunity that entailed moving to Montana, which is often seen as a less progressive venue for healthcare. I respectfully disagree. In the early 1990s we were working in partnership with companies to develop barcoding medication administration for patient safety. The Institute of Medicine report *To Err Is Human: Building a Safer Health System* was published in November 1999. We, along with many others, were advancing patient safety without knowing exactly how far ahead of the curve we were. With the development of the systems of medication administration, there were perpetual questions of why and why not. Before LEAN principles were understood and utilized in the healthcare specctrum, workflow analysis was already being done. It was my first introduction to the impact of human factors on quality and safety.

Lesson learned: Do not assume that work in a nonacademic setting is not profound. This work also needs to be shared and published.

Montana's setting made obtaining my master's degree very challenging. I found a new methodology of educational learning through an online venue from an unknown university at the time, located in Phoenix, Arizona. My professors were moonlighting from multiple universities, such as Yale, Harvard, Stanford, and the University of Washington. These experiences with a cohort of diverse learners and educators broadened my passion for innovation. One of the courses I was enrolled in focused on systems thinking and chaos theory. My eyes opened with a new lens of systems thinking, where connections and leverage points influenced quality improvement and patient safety.

I moved into executive roles as the senior vice president for quality and patient services, corporate compliance officer, and chief nursing officer (CNO). In those roles, I continued to challenge the status quo. In one executive medical staff meeting, leaders of the physicians held the argument that quality care was being provided by our service line of women's and children's care. *I* held the perspective that the cesarean section rate was too high for our level of service. The medical staff leaders felt that the care met national average rates. *I* felt, in essence, that I was politely being told to stand down on this quality issue. I leaned into my training on influencing. Influencing with data is one tactic, but bringing in the human face through storytelling is another. Then I asked the simple question, "Can we look each other in the eye and say with 100% confidence that we have nothing more to do to improve quality?" Silence filled the room—it was the start of novel discussions and more dedicated actions to ensure continuous initiative toward the greatest performance of safety and patient care.

Lesson learned: Quality, innovation, and transformation never sleep. Create a culture that is transparent and willing to learn perpetually.

My Magnet-designated hospital would dance in pink gloves for breast cancer awareness in 2009, introducing the era of social media infancy for healthcare. There was a genuine lack of understanding regarding the impact that social connections would have on individuals through this global platform. The video went viral—people vacationed in our city to see the pink glove hospital, and suddenly hospitals were making videos showing their employees in humanistic, fun venues. Our hospital showed healthcare in a fun, healing setting and openly displayed the many powers these connections had. The video also connected me with the company that manufactured the gloves. My thirst for human-centered product designs met a company that was willing to explore how products could support nursing practice. Finally, an opportunity was being given to design a product embedded with EBP. Products designed to ensure standardization and reduction of variation, ultimately advance patient safety.

In 2014, I joined Medline Industries, Inc., as the CNO. I stepped out of the world of healthcare delivery that I had known for all of my career, and entered the world of healthcare product manufacturing. My thinking expanded from "why", to "what if"? "What if a scale was designed to assist in self-management of congestive heart failure (CHF) through human behavior science and visual cuing?" I worked with a team of engineers, patent attorneys, and product managers to fine tune the design I had envisioned. The heart saver scale is my first patent approved by the patent office.

Lesson learned: It takes partnerships to get an idea developed into a prototype and eventually into a product to be used in the market. Network and develop partnerships beyond the hospital.

I love the brilliance I see within nursing, yet nursing often fails to recognize its own intellectual property. My intellectual property has value and so does yours.

SUPPLEMENTAL RESOURCES

- American Nurses Association Foundation
  https://www.nursingworld.org/foundation
- Certified Nursing Aide
  nurse.org
- Institute of Medicine. (2000). *To err is human: Building a safer health system.* Washington, DC: National Academies Press.
  http://www.nationalacademies.org/hmd/~/media/Files/Report%20Files/1999/To-Err-is-Human/To%20Err%20is%20Human%201999%20%20report%20brief.pdf
- Systems Thinking
  thesystemsthinker.com
- Chaos Theory
  https://www.ncbi.nlm.nih.gove/pmc/articles/PMC2465602
- The Era of Social Media Infancy for Healthcare
  https://www.ncbi.nlm.nih.gov/pmc/articles/PMC4103576
- The Story of The Pink Glove Dance
  https://oregon.providence.org/our-stories/t/two-years-later-the-pink-glove-dance-still-moves
- How to Obtain a Patent
  https://www.usa.gov/features/eight-steps-to-patent-your-invention

My Roadblocks Were Simple Redirections to the Path I Was Meant to ~~Take~~ Blaze!

BOBBI MARTIN, MSN, RN

"The world's health depends on nursing, and the possibilities to impact global health are limitless if we view them in the ongoing lens of hope."

I grew up in Youngstown, Ohio, a steel town, blue collar in every way. Although education was valued by my mom, and I was expected to do well in school, college wasn't in the plan. My mom, brother, and I were poor, if you were to categorize us by income. However, my mom was a pioneer. She raised me through charity work with the Ohio Bell Telephone Company Pioneers. We collected and distributed food, clothing, shoes, and toys for children; fed elderly residents in nursing homes; and spent every holiday celebrating with pediatric residents at her favorite handicapped children's home. This charity work was nothing remarkable, it was simply something we did.

I knew organically that I was a disruptor, before it was ever such a thing. In high school, I quit cheerleading, gymnastics, and track to find authentic, meaningful circles. Soul searching, and the death of three of my four closest friends in a car accident my senior year, steered me to a small town. I lived in a farmhouse without a TV, phone, or stereo, and I went to nursing school. I continued to quietly find my way without distraction in the solitude of my little farmhouse. I was more present in each day and in my studies than I had ever been in my life. Hocking College had a 2-year program; year 1: Licensed Practical Nursing, and year 2: Registered Nursing, after a mandatory 6-month work prerequisite. Six students were selected to be exempt from the work requirement. I was one of the six.

The disruption continued. I refused to wear my nursing cap to clinical, and was promptly sent home, yet continually asked why everything was done the way it was, and continued to challenge every status quo. From challenging the culture of standing up so physicians could sit down, to advocating for pain medicine for patients dying with cancer, there was no shortage of trips to the head nurse's office for insubordination during my tenure in the hospitals; nor were their shortages of trips to my dean's in academia. My good friend Ruth Gallagher, PhD, RN, has kept my council throughout my career; and even when I was certain *I* was the problem, that *my behavior* was a pattern that consistently made me *persona non grata* during my employ, she reminded me that I only say what everyone in the room is thinking.

I knew nursing was continually changing, and that I would be forever learning. Clearly naïve, I was certain everyone in healthcare embraced this same quest for knowledge. After one year of nursing as an LPN, and then one additional year as an RN, in a small rural hospital in Southeastern Ohio, I joined Children's Hospital in Columbus, Ohio. It was the height of the AIDS epidemic, pediatric patients were the largest population with HIV, and Marie Manthey introduced us to primary nursing. It was a terrifying, yet an exciting time in healthcare for nurses. We began to lead cooperative-organized care delivery.

I was exposed to the latest evidence-based practice (EBP) standards in the country, and affiliated with the esteemed Ohio State University. After 2 years, I found myself in charge of Children's Hospital's Level 1 trauma center at the pinnacle of my clinical career, while I also finished my bachelor's of nursing degree. Innovation seems commonplace today, but at the time, it was uncharted territory, yet innovation and disruption were all we seemed to do then! We perfected pediatric cardiovascular surgeries, saved premature babies with appropriately sized equipment unavailable just months prior, and functioned like a well-oiled machine. We were a cohesive, collaborative, and respectful team of physicians, nurses, technicians, respiratory therapists, child life specialists, chaplains, firefighters, and paramedics in the beginning stages of a framework that would become a model for interprofessional collaboration and teamwork.

At the time, I continued to work in pediatric emergency at All Children's Hospital in St. Petersburg, Florida, working night shift on weekends, and eliminating my need for a babysitter for my two daughters. In 1998, I experienced yet another devastating loss. The close friend who had survived the first accident in high school died in a motorcycle accident. This experience, nearly 15 years to the date from the first accident, left me unmoored and looking for purpose. Then, in April 1999, two adolescents shocked the world at Columbine High School in Colorado. As an ED nurse, I was compelled to try to stop kids from shooting. I heard myself say, "Someone has to do something!" As a response, I founded Envision Learning Corporation in May 1999, a 501(c)(3) nonprofit organization. This was my first step toward healing, and my first endeavor at entrepreneurship. While launching Envision, I earned my master's degree in nursing education in order to be better equipped to teach adolescents and adult learners, and finally, to understand curriculum design.

At Envision, cadres of dedicated, emergency pediatric nurses and student resource police officers teamed up to provide 10-week conflict resolution programs for first-time adolescent offenders. We would meet at police substations in underserved neighborhoods, and work with teens and their parents to keep them out of trouble. We maintained an 87% nonrecidivism rate, and our team volunteered throughout Pinellas County schools to provide violence prevention education to high-risk students.

After 20 years as a pediatric emergency night shift nurse, coordinating Envision Learning Corporation for 5 years, and raising a family, I joined the ranks of academia. I taught pediatrics and critical care at the local community college, and naturally migrated toward further education. I was accepted to the PhD program of the College of Public Health at the University of South Florida. Because of my life and ED nursing experience, my research interest was adolescent resilience.

As I taught high-risk kids who were first-time offenders, I saw the impact and influence of having a low socioeconomic status, which I had personally experienced as a child. I wanted to understand why I was able to overcome my circumstances and contribute to society successfully, while many others in similar lower socioeconomic environments could not. Through my years of research, I found that the two most important and consistent characteristics for resilience in children, besides having an average intelligence, are the expectation placed on a child's behavior and performance (which may not necessarily come from the parent), and, overwhelmingly, a feeling of hope. Resilient children are those who can see beyond their current circumstances, and instead, *see what could be.* That was my mindset in Youngstown, and now in nursing.

While pursuing my research, I had a consistent rotation teaching at a 220-bed local hospital with endless opportunities for improvement. I was approached by the CNO and head physician of the cardiovascular team. They wanted a director of nursing who could raise the level of nursing care to match the level that was being observed when my nursing students were working on different hospital units. The leadership team identified that I had cultivated an engaged workforce and a collaborative learning environment, through training I was able to provide with my students. They invited me to become the assistant CNO to replicate that collegial learning environment in the workplace.

Eager to elevate the performance of nurses at the bedside, and thinking I could make a much larger impact on the nursing workforce, I took the job. I was challenged with new problems: higher acuity patients, staffing shortages, knowledge and experience shortages, poor skill mixes, and technology that was intended for safety, but hindered efficiency. Often, what was meant to increase safety, promoted unsafe practices and shortcuts. Within months, the big picture became clear. I realized the enormity of the academic-to-practice gap: rapid technological improvements, attention paid to the patient experience, and a shift to value-based care and quality patient outcomes.

I'd read Berkow, Virkstis, Stewart, & Conway's (2009) article that indicates nearly 90% of nurse educators think their graduates are ready to safely practice, versus the 10% of hospital administrators who believe this to be true, and after the longest year of my executive life, I knew it was true. I returned to academia to identify the primary gaps between what was taught, what was practiced, and what were the latest EBP standards.

As a novice faculty member, I taught students at a level they could only aspire to be, an expert one, but left out fundamental basics that needed to be reinforced and validated, such as handwashing. As I grew and refined my understanding, I moved into roles where I could drive home EBP standards. I became a program director, assistant dean, and dean for one of the largest nurse educators in the United States. I continued to struggle to close the gap through academia. I was selected to participate in Johnson & Johnson's Campaign for Nursing's Future Faculty Leadership and Mentor Program and received the National League of Nurses Health Information Technology grant in 2009.

However, I felt I was missing a key element of the picture: the actual Transition to Practice process. I joined a leading U.S. company that pioneered nurse residencies after the publication of the Institute of Medicine's seminal report, *The Future of Nursing: Leading Change, Advancing Health* (2011). For two years, I became part of the inner workings of hospitals, ranging in many different sizes, which built the foundation, through research and EBPs, for the Transition to Practice programs utilized in the United States.

Finally, I knew what to do. I approached the president of the college I had previously been affiliated with, and asked him to support an incubator company dedicated to supporting *nurses in transition* with evidence and training that was just-in-time. It would not only improve nurse competency, satisfaction, and retention, but would improve patient outcomes. As executive director of this new company, I developed an online learning and benchmarking platform that closed the academic-to-practice gap among U.S. nursing school graduates. The platform became so successful, it was acquired by one of the largest hospital groups in the United States.

Just before the acquisition, a young boy named Patrick had been suffering from a congenital heart condition in his hometown of Jinja, Uganda. Patrick was flown to the United States for treatment. Unfortunately, the condition had taken its toll on Patrick's small body and he died soon after arriving. Patrick's sister had a similar heart condition, and she and her mom returned to the United States for what became a successful surgery and outcome. She was accompanied to the United States by the chief executive officer and the chief medical officer of Whisper's Magical Children's Hospital in Patrick, and his sister, Gift's, hometown. Both leaders held that the most important need they have is education. Within 2 months, all the nurses and physicians at Whisper's Children's Hospital in Uganda had access to the latest EBP-learning modules I developed, and I was on my way to Uganda to learn about their work, to collaborate, and to share up-to-date knowledge about pediatrics.

What has seemed like chance happenings throughout my career, have culminated with the creation of Global Nurse Network (GNN). GNN's vision is to sustain and support well-being and care delivery worldwide. Our mission is to globally connect expert nurses to practicing nurses, instantaneously, for the betterment of the health of our communities. We use a learner's mindset, and work alongside our healthcare delivery partners and patients to learn their needs and wants. This process is instrumental in the co-creation of ideas driving the development of new intentional teaching models and execution.

Going back to my roots and my undeniable sense of hope, I can say I agree with Cornel West when he says, "I'm a prisoner of hope" (Smith, 2006, p. 160). He says hope is different from optimism, "Hope looks at the evidence and says, it doesn't look good at all. Doesn't look good at all. Gonna go beyond the evidence to create new possibilities based on visions that become contagious to allow people to engage in heroic actions always against the odds, no guarantee whatsoever. I am a prisoner of hope" (Smith, 2006, p. 160). The world's health depends on nursing, and the possibilities to impact global health are limitless if we view them in the ongoing lens of hope.

SUPPLEMENTAL RESOURCES

- Nationwide Children's Hospital. Columbus, OH
  https://www.nationwidechildrens.org
- Johns Hopkins All Children's Hospital. St. Petersburg, FL
  https://www.hopkinsallchildrens.org
- College of Public Health at the University of South Florida
  https://health.usf.edu/publichealth
- National League of Nurses Grants and Scholarships
  http://www.nln.org/professional-development-programs/grants-and-scholarships
- Whisper's Magical Children's Hospital
  http://www.whisperorphans.org/US
- Global Nurse Network
  https://globalresearchnurses.tghn.org

The Winding Road to Caring for the Vulnerable and the Profession

JOYCE M. KNESTRICK, PHD, RN, FNP-BC, FAANP

"The road ahead was not sturdy, but I stayed determined to make a difference in my life, the life of my children, my patients, and the nursing profession."

When I graduated from high school, young women were basically given few options: teacher, nurse, hairdresser, secretary, or bookkeeper. It was the mid-1970s and, in my mind, it was time for women to move away from traditional roles and pioneer in other areas. Even though I considered nursing since caring for my ailing grandmother, I could not see myself in a starched blue *dress* and a white cap. Even worse, my father refused to sign any papers for college and insisted it would be best to find a good husband. Times have changed since the 1970s, and most people today have forgotten about the way women were viewed and treated then. My story is not only a reflection on my experience as a woman, but also a reflection of the change in the profession of nursing over the past 40 years. My journey in nursing has been like traveling on a winding road.

Despite my father's objections, I decided that I would attend college to be a scientist and pursue a degree in chemistry. Timing is not my best suit; many of the chemical companies in my area were closing just before I graduated, so jobs in the chemistry field were hard to find. I ended up in a management position in the retail health food chain where I was employed as a student. I continued to hope that I would have the opportunity to move into a chemist role in the quality improvement division at some point. However, I married and became place bound. Retail management requires long hours, and as I moved to become a district manager, more time and travel were required. After my first child was born, I decided to try being a stay-at-home mother. When my second child was 2 years old, my husband lost his job and my world was drastically changed. While working in retail, many of my customers would tell me that I would make a great nurse, so I started to think about nursing. At the same time, nursing was changing; students could even wear pants! After reviewing several options, including: becoming a teacher, a medical technologist, and an advanced chemistry degree, I switched my sights on nursing. I have not looked back since.

Reflecting on my educational experiences, I might have chosen a different path, but I wanted to move quickly in order to help support my family. So, I enrolled in an associate degree program at the Community College of Allegheny County, Pennsylvania. Since I had my chemistry degree and dual biology major, I advanced to the nursing courses. I had excellent clinical experiences and mentors in that program. During preparation for clinical time, I met a woman who had a black bag full of instruments. I thought she was a physician, but she seemed different. I began to talk with her, and learned that she was a nurse practitioner (NP) who was working with a physician who was losing his vision. She explained the role to me, and although I was focused on finishing school, I always kept the notion of an NP in the back of my mind.

My practice as an RN was interesting, because, again, my timing was always off, and there was an overabundance of RNs in the country at that time, so positions were hard to find. I started to practice at a skilled long-term care facility where I was in charge of over 300 patients on night shift, and was often the only RN on site. This was quite a learning experience. Next, I made a complete turnaround from long-term care to practice at a tertiary care hospital in West Virginia. This transition to tertiary care was a learning curve, but I was up to the challenge, and endeavored to learn all that I could from that experience. The road ahead was not sturdy, but I stayed determined to make a difference in my life, the life of my children, my patients, and the nursing profession. The desire to move ahead in my career prompted me to explore master's degree programs, but that required first completing a BSN despite my BS in chemistry.

I enrolled in a BSN program at Wheeling Jesuit University and completed my BSN. The drive to West Virginia was difficult to manage with two small children, so I decided to take a position at the local community hospital. What an eye-opener! Moving from a relatively autonomous and respected role in the tertiary care hospital to the community hospital, where the nurses still gave the physicians a chair and brought coffee, was almost unimaginable. I told some of my nursing colleagues that I wanted to be an NP, and they pretty much scoffed at my ideas. However, I managed to survive in the environment, gained experience in critical care, and became an assistant nurse manager. I served as a change agent, which is not always welcomed in health systems.

The year my third child was born, I started my master's program. I had planned to be a nurse administrator, but my mentor, Mona Counts, PhD, CRNP, FAANP, FAAN, told me I was going to be an NP. My days in my associate program rushed to my mind, as I remembered my encounter with the first NP I met and her little black bag. So, the road turned back to meet me, and I learned to take opportunities when presented.

I moved from the management position to the school of nursing and began my experience as a nurse educator, while I put my new NP credentials to use practicing in a clinic caring for patients with Medicaid. Soon after, I started my PhD program, and I also practiced with Dr. Counts in a clinic she established on her back porch. Eventually I became a nurse educator and started an FNP program in a small college in West Virginia, while still practicing in a clinic that served the underinsured. My desire to help others, particularly the most vulnerable in the community, were coming full circle.

Dr. Counts and I continued to manage an NP-run clinic that expanded to a house, and eventually to a new building. We had over 8,000 patients and provided much needed care to vulnerable patients in mid-Appalachia. The clinic eventually became part of a Federally Qualified Health Center (FQHC), Mona retired, and I continued in my educator role and practice at the clinic for the underinsured. My educator role also took some new twists and turns. I left the program I started and became the Associate Dean of Academic Affairs in an online nursing program, and later the Director of Distance Education at Georgetown University. The opportunity to mentor new nurses and NPs was a way to continue to promote the profession.

I recently served as the president of the American Association of NPs. I believe that my tenure as president has made a significant difference in showcasing the excellent, high-quality, cost-effective care that NPs bring to the healthcare system, and addressing the needs of patients seeking primary care. My timing was finally right. Sometimes the road to making a difference is a winding one. Sometimes you are called to do something, and you do not always answer the call. When you answer the call, be a servant leader, take command, and follow the road ahead. For me, from chemist to NP, it has certainly been a road worth traveling.

SUPPLEMENTAL RESOURCES

- AANP: *The Voice of the Nurse Practitioner®*
https://www.aanp.org/about/about-the-american-association-of-nurse-practitioners-aanp/historical-timeline

- Frontier Nursing University
https://frontier.edu/family-nurse-practitioner

- Federally Qualified Health Center
https://www.fqhc.org

- Georgetown University, School of Nursing and Health Sciences
https://nhs.georgetown.edu

- Goolsby, M. J., & Knestrick, J. M. (2017). Effective professional networking. *Journal of the American Association of Nurse Practitioners, 29*(8), 441–445. doi:10.1002/2327-6924.12484

- Knestrick, J. M., & Counts, M. M. (2012). Developing a nurse practitioner-run center for residents in rural Appalachia. In M. de Chesnay, & B. A. Anderson (Eds.), *Caring for the vulnerable: Perspectives in nursing theory, practice and research* (3rd ed., pp. 357–364). Burlington, MA: Jones & Bartlett.

- Resick, L. K., Knestrick, J. M., Counts, M., & Pizzuto, L. K (2013). The meaning of health among mid-Appalachian women within the context of the environment. *Journal of Environmental Studies and Sciences, 3*(3), 290–296. doi:10.1007/s13412-013-0119-y

- Hunt, D. D. (2018). *The New Nurse Educator: Mastering Academe* (2nd ed.). New York, NY: Springer Publishing Company.

Innovation—It's Like Riding a New Roller Coaster

NANCY M. ALBERT, PHD, CCNS, CHFN, CCRN, NE-BC, FAHA, FCCM, FHFSA, FAAN

"OFTEN, THE FIRST, AND MANY MORE, IDEAS ARE MISTAKES OR FAILURES THAT NEED TO BE DISCARDED IN ORDER FOR THE INNOVATOR TO ACHIEVE SUCCESS IN THE FUTURE."

When I think about my innovation journey, the words that come quickly to mind are exhilaration, fun, growth, and inspiration. These words transformed over time and were not so pretty at first, but improved as my project continued to make progress.

I was a clinical nurse specialist working among a team of other clinical nurse specialists involved in cardiovascular care at a large, Midwest medical center of excellence. The clinical nurse specialist role was a perfect match for me, as it allowed for creativity and my boss was open to possibilities. She had a vision that clinical nurse specialists could make change happen, and was proud of our previous successes. One of my three areas of expertise was heart failure. Plans were made to open a new heart failure ICU that would be separate from the coronary care unit. To my knowledge, other hospitals had telemetry, progressive care, or nonmonitored heart failure units, but not ICUs specifically for one cardiac population. At the time, we still did not have a lot to offer patients with heart failure—an angiotensin-converting enzyme inhibitor, beta-blocker, digoxin, and loop diuretic, were the cook-book primary therapies for ambulatory and stable-hospitalized patients. And, when critically ill, we placed a pulmonary artery catheter, and used intravenous vasodilator (nitroprusside), inotropic agents (dobutamine, dopamine, and milrinone), and diuretics to reduce systemic vascular resistance, improve left ventricular pump function, and facilitate diuresis, respectively.

Our nurse manager was worried that we would have a hard time getting nurses to want to work in an intensive care setting that did not look and feel like a typical ICU. Yes, patients had central intravenous lines and were hemodynamically monitored. Yes, there were intravenous medications that needed to be titrated, but most patients were awake and alert and did not resemble the intubated, sedated, cardiogenic shock patients that our coronary care unit received.

I am not sure where I came up with the idea; really, I think it just kind of popped into my head and I couldn't just shove it aside. I started thinking that one way to get nurses to love working in the unit was to allow them to practice autonomously. I imagined that a physician (there were no advanced practice providers back then) would place an order for an intravenous vasodilator and/or an inotropic drip, and nurses would titrate the drip based on the mean arterial pressure, without waiting for individual orders to titrate. I envisioned that once an order was written to down-titrate an intravenous drip and discontinue, that nurses could work autonomously to make that happen, without having to make phone calls to obtain specific orders during each step of the program plan. Once the intravenous vasodilator or inotropic therapies were discontinued, and the physician wrote an order for an angiotensin-converting enzyme inhibitor or hydralazine + nitrate therapy (for patients with moderate-to-severe renal dysfunction) at the lowest dose, I pictured that nurses could automatically up-titrate the dose to the target dose using a preprinted algorithm. There would not be a need for individual orders. Once I had those thoughts running around in my head, I expanded the plan to include up- and down-titration of all routinely used heart failure therapies based on algorithms that would be designed.

When the program plan was in place, I approached the physician who was the department head for our heart failure and transplantation service line. He loved the idea, which gave me a feeling of euphoria. I had an idea that looked to be feasible. It was novel, and it forced me to think in a new way. Since the program plan needed to be rigorous enough to be operational in clinical practice, I set myself up for the challenge of figuring out how to make it work. Challenges have always been fun to me, so I was in my element.

The next step was the work of developing the many algorithms and pocket cards that made up the program. Of course, I wanted to ensure patient safety as a top priority, and that nurses would feel comfortable taking the steps needed to get patients from a starting dose of a medication to the target dose. Or, in the case of an oral diuretic, that patients were on a dose to create euvolemia, not hypovolemia. Hours were spent in developing and then revising the algorithm, to the tune of about 6 months of work, much of which was on my days off or in the evenings. I wanted to "see" the finished product and couldn't seem to take a break until it was finished. After multiple tweaks of the plan, and multiple versions of each algorithm, it was time to create individual pocket cards. In high school, I was an art student and this part of the work was pure fun. Moving content around on a page to create white space, and using color, font size, italics, and bold font to bring words forward and catch the eye of the reader, was relaxing and amusing. This part of the plan was smooth. Finally, I was ready to share my work with the department head. He gave his full support to move forward and set up a department meeting for us to discuss the plan with 13 other heart failure cardiologists that made up the team.

When entering the meeting room to discuss the program plan, I had an extra step in my walk, a mix of enthusiasm and apprehension. What would the physicians think? Would they allow nurses to determine up- or down-titration decisions without an actual discussion with the heart failure fellows at every step of change? Would they think the program was too aggressive? Not aggressive enough? When entering the meeting room, it felt like the birthing of a baby, and I was completely unsure what to expect. Because of the hours of mental equity in the project, I was also somewhat nervous to participate in the discussion. It was important to listen to their views, but I wanted to shield my heart, knowing the effort it took to get to the present state.

So, the meeting gets started and the department head introduces the program. The first physician who spoke up once the department head asked for feedback stated, "I don't like it and I'm not going to use it." If I could have found a black hole to slip into, that is what I would have done. Instead, my head went down and I waited for the next shoe to drop. But surprise, surprise, the department head challenged the group by saying, "You are going to use it and here is why. ..." Honestly, I cannot even remember the rest of his words, except that he discussed timely, 24/7 management, and discussed that we needed to be leaders, not followers in improving patient outcomes. When he ended his comments, another physician began discussing his experience at another medical center, where an extubation protocol was implemented that allowed ICU nurses to wean patients from the ventilator and extubate, all with one order to begin the protocol. The protocol did not cause harm, and nurses loved having the autonomy to do the right thing. Then, a third physician spoke out about another protocol that was completed at his previous hospital related to heparin drips and maintaining activated clotting times. By the end of the meeting, the team consensus was to give the plan with all the algorithms a try; some team members remained silent, but they did not voice dissent.

After the roller coaster ride of excitement, then despair, then renewed energy that occurred during the department meeting, I wanted to share the good news with colleagues and provide them with some details of the novel program. My excitement must have resonated in my voice, as we had never had a program that matched what I was developing. At the time, I honestly don't remember receiving cues from my colleagues that they did not like the plan. However, at my next one-on-one meeting with my boss, she told me to "watch my back," that my colleagues had spoken to her about my plans, and that they had concerns. She also told me that she spoke to the department head, who loved the new program, and because of that, she would allow me to continue. The message to "watch my back" felt like a painful shock and it made me wonder who and how many colleagues did not like the program? I had never been in a position before where my colleagues had something to say about my work, but not able to say it to me directly. The renewed energy deflated somewhat, and I had to make choices regarding next steps. I chose to quietly continue on my path to bring the project forward. Communication among my physician colleagues, pharmacy colleagues, nurse manager, and boss stakeholders continued, but silence prevailed as the work continued.

Fast forward to months later when we unveiled the program plan. The nurses loved it and so did the physician team (attending physicians and heart failure fellows-in-training). I spent a lot of time in the unit conducting detailed daily rounds to ensure that the algorithms were used as designed, and that nurses felt adequately trained to make the best decisions possible. And, yes, nurses were proud of the increase in autonomy they had in making decisions about patient care in the unit, especially when they received attaboy feedback from the medical team, who were happy to see patients progress, without the need for multiple phone calls. In the next 2 years, we had over 50 site visits from hospitals who wanted to learn about the program. That was an extremely fun and rewarding time for me—to share our work, meet new colleagues in heart failure, and learn through the questions asked at the meetings. And, to come full circle, the physician who stated he was not going to use it became a big supporter of the program and would discuss it at national forums.

To date, over 22 years later, the algorithms are still in use by nursing caregivers in the heart failure ICU, although they've gone through edits and changes, as new knowledge of heart failure and new therapies became available. In addition, the State Board of Pharmacy changed state policies on medication delivery, limiting the use of some of the original algorithms. In the end, my first innovation was important to others and personally fulfilling to me.

Before concluding, I want to leave you with the lessons I learned from this first foray into innovation at the workplace, as I was lucky that my first visualization of the program was accepted by leaders who ultimately made decisions about its use and viability. Often, the first, and many more, ideas are mistakes or failures that need to be discarded in order for the innovator to achieve success in the future.

- Innovation is fun AND work. Expect to spend your own time developing and massaging your innovation. It is not likely that all the pieces will fall into place immediately or that paid work time will be given to develop and cultivate your ideas.

- Think of innovation like a large puzzle that you need to put together. You know the pieces will all fit eventually, but you need to be patient with the process and watch the "picture" emerge.

- Seek collaborators who have your back; those who want you to succeed and can cheer you on when the going gets tough. It is okay to receive criticism, as the criticims could ultimately spur changes that improve the innovation, or increase its feasibility, scope, or usability.

- Show your excitement to people who want to listen. Develop your elevator speech and practice your delivery, so that when it counts, you will be ready to "talk the talk" with the right cadence and emphasis.

- The more novel your innovation is, the more skepticism you may receive. Listen to feedback, but stay focused on your vision. It is hard for some people to grasp what they cannot imagine or see. It is even harder for some to see value in an innovation that is the first of its kind, regardless of it is a device, gadget, process, or algorithm. Remain the cheerleader and push forward.

- Once implemented, diffusion of innovation takes time. Be prepared to spend time ensuring overall success. You are the expert and your knowledge will be valuable to the innovation's adoption.

- Do not be afraid to divorce yourself from the innovation when the time is right. As we know, change is constant, so new ideas will emerge. Be proud that you set the stage for future nurse innovators.

SUPPLEMENTAL RESOURCES

- Reed, P. G., & Shearer, N. B. C. (2018). *Nursing knowledge and theory innovation: Advancing the science of practice* (2nd ed.). New York, NY: Springer Publishing Company.
- Melnyk, B. M., & Raderstorf, T. (2020). *Evidence-based leadership, innovation and entrepreneurship in nursing and healthcare: A practical guide to success.* New York, NY: Springer Publishing Company.

The Nursing Playbook

NANCY NAGER, MSN, RN

"I KNOW THERE'S A SOLUTION TO EVERY PROBLEM AND I KNOW I CAN ALWAYS FIND IT."

There was no revelation or flashbulb appearing above my head. It was a gradual process. Perhaps serendipitous. I started my healthcare career as a candy striper, pinkish red-striped uniforms and all. I have no idea how that happened or why, but it did. I guess becoming a nurse was an early choice, although at that time, choices were limited for women. I went to an all-girls collegiate junior high/high school. They prepared us for college, so I never learned to type or sew or cook; I learned how to study. I loved math and science. I also went to junior achievement, an after-school activity, where you learn about business.

I guess you'd call me a "can-do" person. My only job outside healthcare was decorating cakes at Zayre's; I had no idea how to do that, but I took the job and figured out how to do it after the fact. It has become my life's philosophy. I know there's a solution to every problem and I know I can always find it. So that sets the stage for the story of my career.

I am a nurse, an entrepreneur, a businesswoman, and a supporter for the advancement of women. It is my commitment and passion. I have experienced almost every aspect of healthcare delivery both clinical and administrative. My specialty is behavioral health, having received a master's degree in psychiatric nursing from Boston University. I started my own business in 1990, simply because I was tired of making money for other people who had no idea what they were doing. However, I did have an understanding of clinical innovation that I strongly felt offered a better level of care to my targeted patient population. My approach was nontraditional. I didn't play by the "Harvard business" playbook. I invested in people and encouraged productivity through respect and caring. It is no surprise that by concentrating on people, rather than spreadsheets, you can succeed. But then again, it depends on your goal. Are you in it to grow exponentially and sell, or do you want to make a good living and have a life over the long haul? I chose the latter and regret nothing.

My business began with a desk, a phone, a network of business associates, and a business plan. What counted was the network. Those wonderful few who chose a small piece of my business plan encouraged me to proceed. The business provided behavioral health services to the elderly with a twist. It looked holistically at the individual's needs and promoted a medical/psychiatry approach to care. The elderly are very susceptible to changes in their physical health that are the cause for behavioral manifestations. How often do we see a urinary tract infection (UTI) cause delusions or confusion? At the time, most behavioral health services were driven by a psychology model. Mine was driven by a medical model. It caught on quickly and became a standard level of care as others jumped on. I was previously told that some physicians would never go to long-term facilities to see and treat their elderly residents, but they did.

That model spilled over into 24/7 inpatient medical and psychiatry programs that we developed and managed, and that treated concomitant illnesses simultaneously. An integrated model of care was developed, which was extremely effective and successful, but difficult to manage, and, later on, with changes in reimbursement, more difficult to sustain. Home care and crisis services were added, and then reimbursement became a challenge there as well.

My advice to those in healthcare has always been to keep moving forward, diversify, strategize, and find the next growth engine. Everything changes—reimbursement, technology, competition. Where do you go next? I, later, decided to add medical billing, and wow—it is what brought me to the point where I could sell my company at a high point, and where growth was by no means at an end. It had continuous potential, but my time after 28 years was coming to an end. I wanted to do something else with my experience and background, and perhaps experience less stress (is that possible?).

Currently, I am now back to my roots. I still own and operate a scaled-back behavioral health company focused on the care of the elderly and disabled in outreach locations. I serve on many boards in the public, private, and nonprofit arenas with experience on advisory boards, boards of directors, and boards of trustees. I am the VP/president elect of The Boston Club, a group of 700 women dedicated to the advancement of women in their careers. I am active with Northeastern and Boston University's programming to advance nursing into leadership positions, entrepreneurship, and innovative venues. And, I am proud to be on the board of SONSIEL, my newest adventure that is an exciting opportunity to combine many of my passions and goals that support nursing, advance women, encourage innovation and leadership, and most of all effect change.

Personally, I am a mother, a grandmother, a sister, an aunt, a friend, and a relative. I am an optimist, a can-do person, and a problem-solver. I enjoy all warm weather activities and am not a lover of the cold. I do love to travel, and have been fortunate to do much of it with good friends and relatives—in places where I have met many more good friends. I am beginning a new chapter in my life, having recently lost my husband of 47 years. I call it the year of "firsts". What comes next, is what you make it. I will make it worthwhile.

SUPPLEMENTAL RESOURCES

- Boston University, Nursing Initiatives
  http://www.bu.edu/bunow/tag/nursing
- Northeastern University, School of Nursing
  https://bouve.northeastern.edu/nursing
- The Boston Club
  https://www.thebostonclub.com

Zenventuring Through Business and Life

MICHAEL LAWLER, MSN, BS, RN, FNP-BC, EMBA, MGCP

> *"I HAVE LEARNED TO TRUST MY INSTINCTS ENOUGH TO CARRY*
> *ON WHEN READY AND ABANDON WHEN NECESSARY."*

One evening while working the bar, two of my regular customers, Lenny and Tom, were imbibing their liquor of choice. They were both professional businessmen, which is probably why I choose them to proclaim the following statement, "Gentlemen, I want to do something that helps people." Within 3 months, that simple, yet direct invocation rerouted my life to Delaware and into an RN program, and eventually into an NP (nurse practitioner) program. I was pursuing the certified registered nurse practitioner (CRNP) role from day one, and executed upon that directive with vigor.

In my mind, if I wanted to be an NP, then I had to measure up to a physician, so I studied as one. As I entered the healthcare industry in the fall of 1996, my objective was to absorb as much medical and nursing knowledge as possible. I consumed two physicians digest cassettes each day on my way to work during my 75-minute rides to Masonic Village. While working as a nursing assistant at the hospital, I would tactfully gain entrance into the physician's lounge, and read the discarded journals laying on the break tables. I would visit the libraries of the two local hospitals and the public library, while collecting all the medical journals, audio cassettes, and materials that were left behind, and stored them in my backpack for break time reading.

By 2005, I was plotting the launch of *Angels on Call*, my third healthcare venture. I think it's important to share the moment, or cascade of moments, that ignites the entrepreneurial passion in a person. While treating my patients, I would seek community rehabilitation care services. These services were not readily available, nor were they adequate when delivered. According to my Strengthsfinder analysis, I am an idealist and strategic thinker, among other personality traits. This combination of traits, and the willingness to accept risk, was the lure of entrepreneurship that I couldn't ignore.

When I started my entrepreneurial journey, I didn't know that I could think this way or apply it on demand in critical situations. Frankly, it felt a bit more awkward and off-putting to those around me with whom I shared these thoughts and constructs. I love addressing complex problems. I absolutely drive toward the notion that there is a solution to be discovered. The thought of, "I could do this better!" kept repeating itself through my mind. However, it's easy to see the fixes for problem when you're not in them, and the game of business is pay-to-play— meaning you have to be willing to accept the risk that your solutions may NOT work out. For me, I was willing to accept those risks as my own. Ultimately, all entrepreneurial leaders will have to bet on their own solutions, and accept the possible risk of failure, too. So, I embraced the opportunity and honor to treat people with solutions that derived from my medical and nursing expertise, and recognized that the segue to the business environment was so seductive, that the opportunity to fulfill that mission happened seamlessly for me.

In writing this personalized journey, someone believes I have a story that's worth telling, and for that I am humbled and grateful. I also believe in the exchange of value in relationships. In our world of mutually interactive cooperation and competition, we must both respect and suspect our fellow humans. I do not say this as to conjure up fear and paranoia, but to recognize that we all survive and thrive among one another. For the following writings, I will make a worthy attempt to share my honest and transparent self, in the hopes of cross-pollinating my trials and triumphs for your amusement and future success. And, just like most other stories, this story, my story, highlights the moment where I was called into a gauntlet of achievements and self-discovery, while also enduring precipice-style failures and moments of despair, which eventually led me to earn the incredible treasures that framed my journey.

THE START-UP YEARS 2005-2009

In 2004, the clarity and passion to develop a postacute network started to take root in my soul. I looked at what was available in the marketplace, and by my expectations, it could have been better, much better. I also passionately believe in the ideal, and throughout my story, I will use that as a landmark and an opportunity to deconstruct my experience.

When you share your vision or goals with others, they may not see it as you do, and may even dissuade you from doing it. I have learned to respect and understand those opinions, and incorporate those thoughts and concerns into my vision, if viable. I have learned to trust my instincts enough to carry on when ready and abandon when necessary.

One of the questions I am often asked is, "where did I get the capital from to start the company"? My wife and I only worked part-time, and my other businesses were successful in servicing, but I did not have the business skills to scale, and thusly use these business to my financial advantage. I also did not personally seek money from friends and family, but instead withdrew over $26,000 from various personal credit cards for start-up capital. That's it; the rest of the cash came from retained earnings from operations.

These years were characterized by the molding and forging of my journey as an entrepreneur, my duties, and my dreams. Like many founders, I worked every day with no mention of a "time clock." Angels on Call thrived on customer service by "overpromising and overdelivering." This worked well when I had my hands and thoughts in all details and interactions. I look back at myself during those years with a smirk of incredulity at myself. Our marketing platform and online presence was a significant driver for our growth; our marketing copy and handouts really stood out against our competitors. I would term this period of marketing and advertising as web 1.0. Facebook and Google were not the "monstrosity of advertising and search leads" that they are today, and the idea of hiring a social media manager was a job position yet to be defined.

Those years were a founder's playground. Managing cash flows, developing services offerings, creating and building teams, are certainly the creative zones that keep entrepreneurs focused and awake at 3:14 a.m.—scribbling notes for possible program success points, and motivating speech quips for the troops. It didn't feel like it at the time, but those years meant everything to the future success of the companies, along with the foundations of cash flows, and customer acquisition and retention; an innovative service model was taking shape.

2010-2013: GROWTH WITH A LOT MORE PAPERWORK!

In 2010, Pennsylvania was preparing legislation to certify home health agencies. As an honorable entrepreneur, I had used the lack of certification to my advantage. Angels on Call delivered services on par with skilled nursing representatives, and the partnership with an in-home medical house calls service really added to its credibility. Smaller home care operations lacked organization and processes, and ultimately the fortitude to meet the regulations of Pennsylvania. With the approaching legislation and an introspection of my leadership skills and weaknesses, I was prompted to hire a professional executive director.

There was only one person I could see in that executive position, and she was WAY out of my league in every way. She operated a very well-respected, nationally-owned hospice in Central Pennsylvania; her salary requirements were way above my own pay; and she was due to have her second child by the end of the year. She was introduced to the team as our chief operations officer (COO) in October 2009.

From 2010 to 2013, Honor Healthcare Group became a full-fledged, collaborative operation that had now expanded to four companies: Angels on Call, Housecalls RX, Home Remedy Skilled Nursing, and Legacy Hospice and Palliative Care. There were other companies I started, but some died along the way; most memorable were Heme@Home and Careforall Service Group. But as I have come to accept, companies that do not contribute to your overall strategy are better left for dead, otherwise, you may find yourself resembling them.

These years were characterized by explosive growth in every direction. To my best recall, we had a couple hundred employees, multiple offices, and a commensurate amount of administration. Like most entrepreneurs, administration is a means to an end for great service. But when you are playing with the government's money, paperwork is everything. Gratefully, the COO handled this with absolute integrity and responsibility. To this day, it is one of the behaviors of the companies I am most proud of.

Cash flow was huge and so were the liabilities. I can still vividly recall my wife asking me for a source of $47,000 at 1 a.m. for our initial workers' comp payments due in 10 days. I didn't have an answer for her. Ultimately, we sourced the payment, but I learned to accept the fact that sometimes you just have to go to bed without all the answers.

2013–2015: GROWTH AND THEN THE SALE

By Spring 2013, companies were noticing Honor Healthcare Group and its success. I had an offer to sell in June 2013. It was a very nice number, but I declined. I truly believed that we were building something great, and I wasn't interested in sitting on a beach island just yet. Declining the offer just attracted more top talent to the team, and ultimately a merger with another healthcare group occurred in 2014.

Now that you've gotten a glimpse into my journey, here are four personalized mementos that I would like to share with you that have given me my personally-defined success and peace.

Memento #1: Define your commitment and own it.

In starting Honor Healthcare Group, I evangelized upon two long-term visions that were immutable to me. First, I wanted to reinvent the postacute care network and be recognized on the cover of *Time* magazine for that innovation.

The second vision for Honor Healthcare Group was simple and righteous. Everyone has the right to live and die at home under their own direction and choice. Entering your senior years or disabled-pathway is a return to insecurity, need, and vulnerability. At this time in a patient's life, support systems should be layered, effective, and personalized in aiding someone to determine their remaining life path. I didn't believe the system was trying hard enough to accomplish that goal. I couldn't tolerate the healthcare system directing another 78-year-old individual to leave their home to decline in health, then die.

"Wow! What passion! What commitment!", people would say in response to these zealous labors. Those affirmations were confirmation that I was doing something meaningful. That's the good part; but the payment for such commitment was much more impactful.

I was on call from March 12, 2006, to September 30, 2015, 24/7, 365 days a year for nine-plus years. Families calling with questions, nurses calling for orders, and staff calling for clarity. What do I remember about those years? Running through a Thanksgiving Day 10K race and giving orders to a daughter about how much Roxanol to give to her terminal mother. Taking a call just a few hours after the birth of my third child. Taking off in a plane for Alaska while the call gets disconnected as we ascend to an altitude beyond cell towers. Countless calls from 11 p.m. to 7 a.m. looking for rescue, answers, and medication refills. At that time I just marched ahead with my best effort. Today, I now recognize it all as a part of the *entrepreneur's stress syndrome* and it has taken me a few years to finally and fully decompress from this syndrome, and reset my balance.

What made Honor Healthcare Group so progressive was its reinvention of the postacute healthcare model on multiple aspects. The company was designed to provide solutions to two major pain points for the patient and its stakeholders: healthcare paternalism, and care continuum fragmentation.

This started with putting the patient back at the center of the decision-making pathway in regard to the patient's healthcare. Too many times I saw providers, care managers, and facilities override the patient's life choices in the best interests of that patient's health.

Honor Healthcare Group strategically acquired or built every service for a care continuum model with the patient at the hub, and all services acting as the spokes in their self-defined care pathway.

Utilizing personal ambassadors, 24/7 direct provider communication, an energetic and ambitious communication protocol including all stakeholders, and refocusing our team directive to treat the patient as a person with health problems, versus a disease dictating a person's journey, was our reinvention. Today it may not seem as profound to do practice this way, but it was in 2010.

Services included in-home medical house calls, personal care, skilled nursing and therapy, palliative and hospice care, and inpatient-skilled nursing. And to this day, I am proud to have been one of the first persons to put it all together at a regional scale, even when the managers of Medicare were already pregnant with a nationwide solution—managed care organization.

Memento #2: Stay ahead of the motorcycle!

What does that mean? I ride an adventure motorcycle and a race bike. One of the key techniques riders use to stay safe on the road is the cognitive scheme of staying ahead of the motorcycle in time and space. Think about what's coming your way in terms of near, far, and immediate future. Teaching yourself to act in a moment that has yet to come is a fantastic skill. Simple, but profound.

While I had started other companies prior to Honor Healthcare Group, I didn't know what it meant to be a leader of an organization. What I realized is that, learning to be a leader in the middle of the process, with no prior training, can be both poignantly exhilarating and surgically introspective. As Honor HealthCare Group grew from one, to three, to five companies in 5 years with over 300 employees, I started to recognize that I wasn't fully prepared for this level of leadership. So, in 2012, I opened the discussion with our company's COO at the time, and boldly stated that, "for this organization to continue its trajectory it needs to be with a different leader." With a clear conviction, I rationally and logically determined that the leader of Honor Healthcare Group would, and should, not be me. In 2014, I wholeheartedly supported the transition to a new executive team. In retrospect, I have continued to be confident that it was the right move to ensure the success and growth of all those involved.

In 2015, I enrolled at Villanova University for my executive MBA. It was during those years where I began to understand my strengths and weaknesses as a leader. I pursued that degree for the sole mental reenactment of the prior 9 years; earning my executive MBA was one of the most self-actualizing pursuits I have ever had.

Memento #3: Be willing to bet on yourself, while understanding the risks and rewards.

In 2015, operations were going pretty well. Honor Healthcare Group was developing itself as a serious healthcare organization. Infrastructure spending for that year was at least $276,000, and the teams were starting to really understand the magic in the network delivery. My chief financial officer (CFO) had strategically engineered a loan for launching all of the companies under the Honor Healthcare Group umbrella to new levels of success. To my best recollection, the loan was for approximately $27 million. The contract for this loan was slightly thicker than the Harrisburg city phone book! This was a big number, and one that, to say the least, would be difficult to pay back. Yet, I could only see the value creation and the strategic planning that went into the loan decision of the companies. I signed those loan papers without hesitancy, not that I didn't understand the risk, but I believed my efforts would ultimately overmatch the risk in execution.

A short time later a *black swan* event occurred, and its ripple effect altered the risk and reward balance. As of October 2015, the entire postacute care enterprise now named Honor Health Network would be operated by new owners.

I am often asked how did I feel about the sale when everything seemed to be going so well. My answer is complex and simple. As previously reflected upon, all entrepreneurial leaders are betting on their solutions, and each leader must choose to accept the risk of failure and, at that time, I was ready to accept. For me, I recognized that the risk and reward scale for Honor Healthcare Group was no longer in an acceptable balance.

While I still practice as a family NP today, and stay active in business ventures and start-ups, my full-time focus is on workforce solutions in semi-skilled labor forces. My business partner and I are now on to our next adventure, to reinvent the Business-to-business (B2B), Business-to-company (B2C), and Business-to-employee (B2E) journey and experience in the construction sector.

SUPPLEMENTAL RESOURCES

- StrengthsFinder
  https://www.gallupstrengthscenter.com/home/en-us/strengthsfinder
- Honor HealthCare Group
  http://www.honorhealthcare.com
- Villanova University
  https://www1.villanova.edu/university.html

Be the Change: If It Makes Sense ... Do It

MARY LOU ACKERMAN, MBA, BSCN

"I'VE LEARNED THAT PEOPLE WILL FORGET WHAT YOU SAID, PEOPLE WILL FORGET WHAT YOU DID, BUT PEOPLE WILL NEVER FORGET HOW YOU MADE THEM FEEL."
—MAYA ANGELOU

What do you want to be when you grow up? This is a difficult question to answer at a young age; however, what I know now is that life is a journey shaped by many learning opportunities and experiences along the way. I realized very early in my career as a nurse that there is no end to the possibilities of what can be accomplished when one is willing to challenge the status quo, to learn, and to focus on the impact one can have on people's lives.

What stands out most for me during my career is how important it has been for me to surround myself with smart, passionate people, those who are change makers. Early on in my career, I worked in a community hospital for an inspiring nurse manager who encouraged team work and demanded exceptional client care. She created an environment that expected personalized care, professionalism, and creative problem-solving when faced with challenges. She was happy to listen to any problem as long as you were willing to "own" the solution. She respected, trusted, and supported her nursing staff. In the few years I worked for her, she instilled in me to always challenge the status quo and strive to create great experiences both for clients and colleagues.

Although my "inhospital" experiences began to shape who I would become as a nurse, it wasn't until I took a job as a community nurse at SE Health that I was able to really see and feel the incredible impact nurses can make on individuals and their families. The home care environment required nurses to practice autonomously, tapping into all facets of professional practice. Every patient and their home presented unique challenges/opportunities that had to be addressed in very creative ways. For example, using coat hangers and broomsticks as intravenous (IV) poles, making troughs using garbage bags to wash the hair of a bed-bound patient, and egg cartons to manage medications, are just a few. My creativity skills were constantly being tested; "macgyvering" became a new nursing skill. It was such a rewarding feeling to know you took down a barrier, enabling an individual to remain at home with their loved ones and, even if for just a moment, feel good.

In 1987, I joined the SE Health team of 500 community nurses in Toronto—today we have grown to be a national organization with approximately 10,000 employees led by Shirlee Sharkey, a nurse who is also passionate about innovation. Over the past 30 years, I have held a number of exciting positions, many of which were created out of seeing a need and filling a gap. Back in the early 1990s, we were a very paper-based organization, but at the same time provided care remotely. This meant that everything a community nurse needed to know (schedules, referrals, orders, etc.) had to be read and transcribed over the phone—time consuming, inefficient, and painfully boring. As another example, if someone in the office needed to connect with a community nurse, that person had to start calling each scheduled patient to see whether the nurse was there. Again, time consuming and inefficient. These inefficiencies had to be addressed, as every minute on the phone took away precious minutes to spend with a patient. In addition to my nursing background, I had a hidden passion for technology and took on the role of special projects, implementing a number of game-changing (back in the day) solutions over the years—such as portable fax machines, cell phones, and software to support the automation of manual processes. Tapping into this hidden passion allowed more time for direct patient care, and less time wasted on administrative tasks. By recognizing the need for these changes, I also found the courage and voice to advocate for solutions that would impact patients, clinicians, and the organization.

Building on my passion for community health and my desire to advance care through solving problems with creative solutions, I decided to augment my nursing degree with a graduate business degree (MBA), a unique combination at the time. Advancing my education opened the door to higher level positions of influence within the organization and health system. I spent a few years as the Vice President of Information Management, focused on creating solutions to measure organization performance, and identifying areas of strength to be built on and opportunities for improvement, both internally and externally. This was a pivot point in my career. There were many opportunities to improve patient experiences; however, they were often not within reach inside the walls of our organization. Health system level change was required and not easy to achieve. Collaboration, strategic partnerships, and business model innovation would be the enablers of success.

Today, I am the Vice President of Innovation and Digital Health. Our mandate is to create a future where Canadians can age with agency, dignity, health, and vitality by fostering collaborative, bold thinking through the delivery of digital experiences. The expertise I proudly bring to the team is my clinical background as a nurse, advocating for the patients and their families, and ensuring this future recognizes the incredible impact that nurses have on how these individuals experience life. Over the past couple of years, I have developed a strong network within the health innovation ecosystem. This includes valuable relationships with innovation accelerators, incubators, and many inspiring technology companies to support product development, evaluation of impact, drive adoption, and integration into or transformation of the health system. We have cocreated a digital assistant for older adults who live alone. Using voice technology such as Amazon Alexa, the senior receives a daily check in, medication reminders, and other cuing for events. Based on their responses, if needed, a nurse will do a phone assessment and determine whether one of the 10,000 staff members who work in the area where these individuals live should drop by and address the issues. This solution changes the way home care services are delivered today—from a scheduled visit model, to "just in time" or "right time" visit model, giving the individual peace of mind knowing we are "there when you need us." At an organizational level, it's important to understand how digital tools such as these integrate into clinical workflows to create new service models that create value for individuals, clinicians, and the health system.

In October 2018, we hosted the first ever Canadian EntrepreNurse summit, bringing together nursing leaders from academia, professional associations, and service provider organizations. The key objectives of the summit, and the subsequent action plan, is to enable nurses to have a voice in developing innovation solutions for their patients, families, and healthcare systems, as well as to develop strategies to position nurses as innovation agents. I believe nurses see unmet needs and gaps in care, and have both the vantage and creativity to be innovation leaders. As a nursing leader, I welcome opportunities to mentor the next generation of nurses, helping them to challenge the status quo, seek out solutions, and be a part of health system transformation. I strongly believe that their nursing knowledge of the client journey must lead the way as new solutions are identified and introduced into the health system.

I have had the privilege to spend the vast majority of my nursing career at SE Health and am grateful for all of the opportunity I have had with this progressive organization. Early on in my career, our CEO Shirlee Sharkey (did I mention she is also a nurse), said to me, "if it makes sense, do it." I believe these few simple words gave me the courage to constantly challenge the status quo, find solutions, and make an impact. My top three pieces of advice are:

- Surround yourself with good people;
- If it makes sense, do it;
- Remain humble—partnerships bring strength and new ways of thinking.

Have the confidence and courage to "macgyver" when needed, and embrace your divergent thinking—solutions are within reach, and the future of health is ours to shape.

The Intrapreneurial Nurse

MARGARET A. FITZGERALD, DNP, FNP-BC, NP-C, FAANP, CSP, FAAN, DCC, FNAP

"For me, the characteristic that is most important to nursing is the concept of equality: equal care to all populations with no stratification of care."

Clinician, educator, consultant, author, professional speaker, mentor, advisor, thought leader, business owner, intrapreneur, entrepreneur. These are but a few of the varied roles I have filled as an RN and nurse practitioner (NP). FAANP, FAAN, recipient of three lifetime achievement awards, American Journal of Nursing Book of the Year award, five NP of the Year awards from state and national organizations. These are but a few of the varied accolades I have received. How did a person from a working class family who spent her childhood in public housing and a community college graduate get to this point? It all started by becoming a nurse. Here is what I have learned along the way.

LOOK EARLY ON FOR ROLE MODELS AND OTHER REBEL NURSES

I was fortunate enough to witness the value of nursing at a very young age, which helped to shape my beliefs in this profession from that point forward. I had a close relationship with my aunt who was a public health nurse in Boston, where I grew up. When I was probably only 6 or 7 years old, she would take me out on quarantine rounds with her, as she went around to see patients with infectious diseases and decided whether the family needed to be quarantined, while also providing treatment for these patients. These early experiences greatly influenced me and showed me the power of nursing practice and public health.

REFLECT ON WHY YOU DECIDED TO ENTER INTO NURSING PRACTICE. KEEP THIS IN MIND ALONG THE WAY

Becoming a nurse was an obvious choice, as it melded two of my driving interests: my love of science and my desire to work with people. Throughout my career, I have sought to be an advocate for people and families, and as a family NP, I advocate for best health practices for entire families. This is one reason why I sought the NP role: to have a much higher level knowledge and skill set that would allow me to advocate for and benefit a family in more ways.

STRIVE TO PRACTICE TO THE FULL EXTENT OF YOUR EDUCATION AND LICENSURE

For the RN/NP, it may seem obvious in today's healthcare settings that we should each strive to practice to the full extent of our license, experience, and knowledge base. However, this was not always the case, as RNs and APRNs were once pushed to limit their practice scope and expertise. I found in my earlier days of critical care that those external limits on nursing practice had been, fortunately, moved aside. Our mindset was that we are RNs, we have a very high skill and knowledge level, and to do our best for these critically ill patients, we must practice to the very edge of that knowledge and to the full extent of what is allowable by our license. That's what kept me in critical care for 16 years, prior to becoming a family NP.

LOOK FOR WAYS TO CHALLENGE THE STATUS QUO, WITH INTRAPRENEURIAL PRACTICE

In my years in critical care, I held a variety of leadership positions. A common theme was my constant strive toward being an intrapreneur: a person who started a professional venture within an organized system. I led a group that developed a regionalized approach to interdisciplinary critical care education. I am proud to say that this venture became a national role model. I was also at the forefront of advancing decentralized nursing leadership.

THROUGHOUT YOUR CAREER, ALWAYS LOOK TOWARD YOUR NEXT GOAL

After a successful, varied career in critical care as a staff nurse, I was ready to go to graduate school. Rather than remain in critical care, however, I decided to become a family NP. One of the driving forces in my decision to move on from critical care was my view of the NP role, which was only 20 years into its existence at the time. It was a role that allowed me to advocate for and work with my patients, to work in the community, and to keep people out of the ICU. During my 16 years of working in critical care, I could walk through the ICU many days and see one person after another with what I knew were easily preventable diseases had the patient had access to primary healthcare services. So I left the ICU and began practicing in the community.

I was the first NP to hold a leadership role with an intrapreneurial twist when I set up and opened the first satellite clinic, in the federally qualified community health center. Here, I was able to translate what I had learned in critical care to my new role.

EMBRACE THE BLENDING OF ROLES: INTRAPRENEUR TO ACADEMIC TO ENTREPRENEUR

Among my accomplishments, the one that I am most proud of is creating Fitzgerald Health Education Associates, Inc. When I started it, I did not realize I was starting a company. I was simply trying to fill a void in healthcare. I had entered the academic world, was teaching full time, and was thriving as a university professor. At the same time, I was carrying my intrapreneurial expertise into the university as I started the first family NP program in the city of Boston. I was also asked to help a group of students prepare for the NP boards. At that time, I had taught at the associate, baccalaureate, and master's levels, and I had done a tremendous amount of continuing education teaching. The NP review market was fairly small and the business involved in providing these courses were of the "customer comes to us" model, keeping in mind this was before online education.

While we started small—six students around my dining room table—we quickly evolved into a "we will go to you" model, offering courses across the country and via recordings. That's how we have survived and emerged as Fitzgerald Health Education Associates, LLC. As technology advances, we are able to offer multiple ways of delivering NP review and continuing education live, online, and via MP3. Our company has grown to include 25 faculty consultants who, aside from my work, develop and teach courses. Our product line includes NP and NCLEX® preparation, university courseware, ongoing continuing education for healthcare providers, publications, consultation, and testing.

Have Your Educational Level Match the Work You Do

Another accomplishment of which I am most proud is earning my DNP after two decades of NP practice, and 36 years after entering the nursing profession. I chose to earn my DNP because I had felt during the entire time that I had a master's degree, I was actually doing doctoral-level work, and I had this intense desire to finally be degree-congruent: to hold a degree that matched what I do clinically, what I do in my writing, and what I do in my consulting. The DNP was the way of doing this. Having completed my DNP studies, I finally feel as if my education and professional responsibilities are much more closely matched.

HEALTHCARE EQUITY IS NOT AN OPTION

For me, the characteristic that is most important to nursing is the concept of equality: equal care to all populations with no stratification of care. This, unfortunately, does not exist across healthcare today. The stratification of care that we have in the United States due to issues of poverty, and racial, ethnic, sexual orientation, gender identity, and other factors, prevent many people from accessing high-quality care. Nurses, including NPs, are at the absolute frontline of care, and must carry with us—in the very core of who we are—the ethical concept of beneficence. This is the idea that everybody benefits in the same manner from the healthcare system, and that there is no stratification due to income, ethnicity, sexual orientation, gender, or any other factor. We must be constantly vigilant of those barriers that are thrown in front of us. I have chosen to practice my entire career in a Federally Qualified Health Center (FQHC). I want nurses to realize that practicing in an underserved community is not "just an option" when you can't find a job any place else, but rather this is what you can choose to do, to move along the profession, to move along healthcare in general, and to maximize the overall health of this great nation.

THINK OF YOURSELF AS THE CEO OF YOUR OWN CAREER

I pose a challenge to nurses, particularly those in early career. Think of yourself as the CEO of your own nursing career. What opportunities can you exploit? How can you best direct where your nursing career goes? How can you be that powerful threat?

What I'd like nurses to know that I didn't know earlier is what a fantastic career this can be, if you keep your eyes open and take advantage of every opportunity that is presented to you. I have had at least six, very distinctly different careers in my nearly 50 years as an RN. Each one of them has carried its own challenges, but each one of them has also gleaned tremendous reward.

LOOK FOR THE OPPORTUNITIES TO BE A POWERFUL THREAT

Nurses must keep in mind that only the powerful are a threat. Every pushback to what we do as nurses translates into how our powerful stature is seen as a threat. As exhausting as this can be, we have to recognize this opposition as an impressive statement. If being a threat seems too strong a term to use, recall that you and your nursing colleagues are using your collective power to advocate for patients and your profession. Your nursing background, and your respect for the history and service of our great profession, will surely guide you in your actions.

All RNs and APRNs should be looking ahead to what they can do next with this great career. While you continue to work very hard at maximizing what you can get out of your current experience, also be willing to take a look at what you're going to do next. This will keep your career both novel and interesting. In this way, you will help move ahead all of healthcare, and you will also move ahead the great profession of nursing, and join the ranks of rebel nurses. Be that powerful threat.

SUPPLEMENTAL RESOURCES

- Cash, J. C., & Glass, C. A. (2018). *Family Practice Guidelines* (4th ed.). New York, NY: Springer Publishing Company.
- Fitzgerald Health Education Associates, LLC
  https://www.fhea.com/index.aspx
- Federally Qualified Health Centers
  https://www.fqhc.org/what-is-an-fqhc

The Rebel Nurse's Progress Note

Mentorship, whether informally through a book or podcast, or formally, through an intentional one-on-one connection, is often crucial to seeing your vision become a reality and, ultimately, how you influence the way health and healthcare is delivered. When you're willing to find someone to role model early in your career, it creates a culture of learning and mutual respect. Although there may be setbacks and obstacles along the way, those mentors can be instrumental in how you respond, and is a choice worth considering, as you challenge the status quo. Even nonacademic settings are profound opportunities to seek camaraderie with those who have your back. So, be willing to hear what others have to say and surround yourself with good people.

Also, along your rebel nurse journey, recognize that the road to making a difference is a winding one, but with those twists and turns come the opportunities to diversify, strategize, and grow. Hear what others have to say and consider being open to blended roles that may look different than your expectations. And with every novel idea, every new endeavor, and every innovative thought process, even if you may draw skepticism, be willing to pivot and adapt, no matter the circumstance.

Finally, remain humble as you think about the near, far, and impending future, even when success comes your way. Humility not only gives you a healthy perspective on the sacrifices others may make to support you along the way, it also keeps you motivated in the face of opposition and delay. Because, as one rebel nurse wisely mentioned, once implemented, the diffusion of innovation may take time.

So, as you soak in these words of wisdom from very wise shift disruptors, innovators, and rebel nurses, remember to have limitless hope, as you await the impact your own journey will have on the future of nursing.

> *Who can you surround yourself with that may impart words of wisdom? Consider finding a mentor, as you challenge the status quo.*

Rebel Nurses at the Crossroads: Innovative Methodologies, Reflections, and Resources to Guide the Future of Nursing

Our stories have come to a close, but it doesn't mean the journey is over. As an effort to give you an extra charge and a place to start, this chapter will give you practical methodologies, as well as motivational charges, to achieve an innovative mindset, to find the right team to work alongside in your journey, and to elevate the future of nursing.

The Five "Rights" of Healthcare Innovation

BONNIE CLIPPER, DNP, RN, MA, MBA, CENP, FACHE

"INNOVATION CANNOT OCCUR IN A VACUUM AND SHOULD BE DIVERSE IN THOUGHT AND INPUT."

— BONNIE CLIPPER, THE NURSE'S GUIDE TO INNOVATION: ACCELERATING THE JOURNEY

The idea to write a book about innovation for nurses, *The Nurse's Guide to Innovation: Accelerating the Journey*, was inspired through the many conversations I had while traveling and speaking as the vice president of innovation for the American Nurses Association. There was a common theme in all of these people; they all really wanted to make a difference in the world.

Just like this book you find yourself reading now, *The Nurse's Guide to Innovation* is also written by nurses. And similar to the inspiration behind *The Rebel Nurse Handbook*, after connecting with a host of incredible nurses, who were not only amazing innovators and entrepreneurs but were also fantastic people, the world of nursing seemed to need something "more" as a resource for nurses in the sphere of healthcare innovation. The "more," for the *Nurse's Guide*, was how to move an invention or product in the heads of nurses into the material world, how to create a business plan, how to raise money, and how to get the nurses within their organizations more engaged in innovation, as well as other entrepreneurship and innovation-related conversations.

The knowledge shared in *The Nurse's Guide to Innovation*, and the stories found in *The Rebel Nurse Handbook*, represent an array of experiences and diverse paths through nursing that serve to compliment what you may or may not get in your own nursing journey. In *The Nurse's Guide to Innovation*, our team of authors were inspired to provide guidance and practical tips on entrepreneurship, developing a business or marketing plan, protecting intellectual property, securing financing, or engaging nurses in innovation that will help you advance inventions, ideas, or even enhance engagement in the change process. Both are an inspiring guide for nurses who desire to disrupt the status quo. Both, after several months of these types of conversations, show a commitment to nurses being willing to share their own wisdom to propel other nurses forward into the future of healthcare.

This commitment to seeing nurses specifically advance in the space of innovation, ultimately inspired a methodology that I termed the Five "Rights" of Healthcare Innovation. I'd like to share an excerpt from *The Nurse's Guide to Innovation* here with you that I think explains it best:

> *Innovation cannot occur in a vacuum and should be diverse in thought and input. Just as the Five Rights of Medication Administration (right medication, right patient, right dose, right route, and right time) ensure safety (ISMP, 2007), there should also be five rights to innovation in healthcare. These should include identifying the right problem, settling on the right solution, implementing at the right time, ensuring that the right price allows for scale and sustainability, and ensuring that the right education is rolled out in order to ensure safe and effective rollout. (2019, p. 85)*

BOX 6.1 Five "Rights" of Healthcare Innovation

Right problem
Right solution
Right time
Right price
Right education

SOURCE: Reproduced with permission from Clipper, B., Wang, M., Coyne, P., Baiera, V., Love, R., Nix, D., . . . Weirich, B. (2019). *The nurse's guide to innovation: Accelerating the journey* (p. 85). Cupertino, CA: Super Star Press.

Knowing this piece of insight—whether you recognize it or not—as a nurse, you are an innovator. And I encourage you to take the essence of these *five rights*, and the stories you've read in this book, and start putting them into practice as you disrupt the status quo of healthcare. No matter what season you find yourself in your career, we hope that these resources will inspire you to be the innovative *rebel nurse* that you are!

The Rebel's Innovation Methodology

MARY LOU ACKERMAN, MBA, BSCN

"AN ORGANIZATIONAL CULTURE THAT EMBRACES INNOVATION CELEBRATES THE LEARNINGS THAT COME FROM BOTH INNOVATIONS THAT FAIL AND THOSE THAT SUCCEED."

Innovation is the conversion of great ideas into a desired impact at a specified scale. A methodology is required to effectively go from problem to idea to meaningful impact. Innovation is often a messy process, routinely experienced as two steps forward, one step back. However, a methodology can help take a lot of beta out of the experience, by allowing you to anticipate the pitfalls before you face them, and most importantly by providing insight to when you should continue to move forward and/or learn from your setbacks.

An organizational culture that embraces innovation celebrates the learnings that come from both innovations that fail and those that succeed. In the innovation space it's often said that if you're not failing, you're not innovating hard enough. Not all organizations can embrace failure; therefore, creating a culture that welcomes the failure associated with innovation will enable long-term success. The key is to fail fast and move forward with confidence, knowing that you are doing the right thing. Here are a few things to consider as you actively influence a culture of innovation within your organization.

1.   Clearly define what innovation means within your organization, and what it does NOT mean. What is in scope (product or service areas, geographies, customer groups, process versus business model)? And at what scale of change or impact will you focus your energy (see later discussion of the McKinsey Three Horizons framework, as an example)?

2. Identify who will be the executive sponsor to provide cover when all of the organization's antibodies try to come out and stop the new idea. Ideally, this would be the CEO or someone with equally strong power and "teeth" in the organization.

3. Find innovation champions to be your supporters and advocates throughout the process—they are vital in both the good/easy times, and also the tough times when most people will want to bail.

4. Set metrics that measure both success and failure—a combination of input/process metrics, output metrics, and outcome/impact metrics.

5. As a team: Work out loud, share your stories, ask for their participation in workshops, codesign sessions, and evaluation. This is your core internal team plus your extended external team of partners, customers, and so on. If you're really innovating, you should never have a team that is composed of people from within the four walls of your organization.

6. Build a broader network or ecosystem of partners, both within the healthcare ecosystem and outside it—to strengthen your overall innovation muscle and reach well beyond specific projects.

LET'S GET STARTED: THE MINIMUM VIABLE INNOVATION METHODOLOGY

A minimum viable innovation methodology (MVIM) provides a framework and the tools you can use to achieve success with your innovation efforts. Regardless of the size or scope of the problem you are trying to solve, a framework to guide how you do your innovation work is vital. What differs is the amount of effort/time that will be required to utilize different elements of the framework effectively. This approach was developed by SE Health's Futures team as "our way to work," and can be easily modified to suit your innovations.

The first step to get started: it's important to shape your purpose statement, that is, via a "How might we ... " statement (HMW). This will set the stage and provide clarity as you begin your journey. You will use this HMW statement to challenge the ideas you generate. Are they *really* going to address the purpose? Solve the problem? Are they thinking big enough?

Next, determine what scale of impact or change you are innovating against. Using the McKinsey Three Horizons model, consider that different horizons reflect different degrees of change relative to today and the status quo. These changes are either new capabilities (left axis) or changes in the business model. Mapping your ideas on the three horizons will give you a good sense of the effort and impact you are setting out to make, as described in Figure 6.1.

- Horizon 1: Innovation at the core can sometimes be described as a quality improvement; however, it is innovative if a new capability or change to the business model is introduced.

- Horizon 2: Innovation that reshapes or evolves the core. Often this type of innovation introduces new customers to your offerings, or provides an entrance into new markets.

- Horizon 3: Innovation that disrupts your current offering. The creation of brand new capabilities and business models as a response to external disruptors.

The new capabilities you introduce with the degree of change to your current business model require a different level of focus, effort, resources, and risk tolerance in order to determine your "sweet spot." Innovation teams should determine what degree of their time and

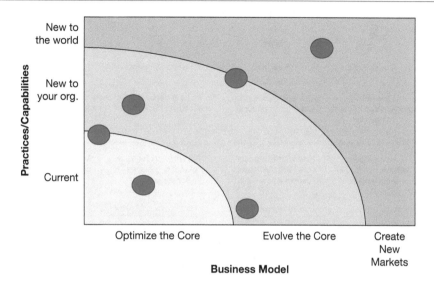

FIGURE 6.1 The McKinsey Three Horizons Model

SOURCE: Adapted from McKinsey Quarterly. (2009). Enduring ideas: The three horizons of growth. Retrieved from https://www.mckinsey.com/business-functions/strategy-and-corporate-finance/our-insights/enduring-ideas-the-three-horizons-of-growth

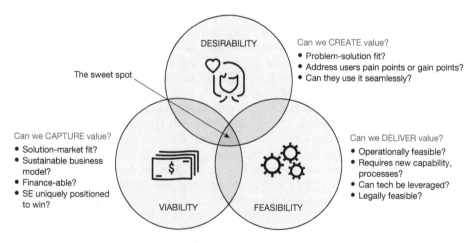

FIGURE 6.2 The "Sweet Spot" of Innovation

SOURCE: Copyright 2019 Saint Elizabeth Healthcare.

**Adapted from IDEO design thinking

resources they want to spend in each horizon as they lay out their priorities. This spot envelops desirability, viability, and feasibility: Is our idea desirable? Do our stakeholders want a solution like this? Is it feasible? Can we really make this happen? And finally, is it viable? Should we do this? Is there enough value that we are offering?

Linking back to your purpose statement described earlier is critical as you work through the process to find that "sweet spot." Let's dive into it a little deeper (Figure 6.2).

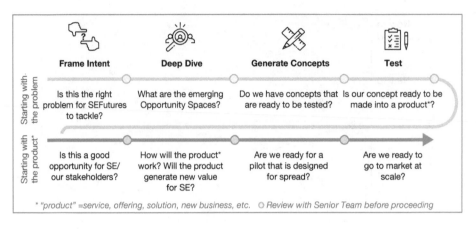

FIGURE 6.3 Saint Elizabeth Futures Innovation Model

SOURCE: Copyright 2019 Saint Elizabeth Healthcare.

Desirability: What problem are we solving? What value are we creating? Are we addressing current pain points? Are we introducing new risks? What could be the unintended consequences?

Viability: What do we anticipate the return on investment to be? Is there a market fit for this solution? Is our organization uniquely positioned to win in this space?

Feasibility: Do we have the knowledge, skills, and resources to offer this solution? Are there new capabilities required to ensure our success? What barriers might we face?

The amount of effort one puts into truly understanding these three areas will impact the likelihood of success or at the very least minimize the amount of resources utilized, when the decision is made to stop moving forward and learn from the experience.

Finally, a step-by-step innovation methodology outlines four key phases to take, in order to go from problem or idea to validated solution—ready to implement at scale—while always keeping your purpose statement HMW front and center. This phased methodology helps your team and other stakeholders clearly understand what types of questions need to be answered at each stage of the innovation process (Figure 6.3).

At its highest level, this innovation framework is made up of four phases that can either start with the problem we are trying to solve (top line) or start with the new product idea (bottom line). Each phase starts and ends with what we like to call a "point of commitment" (note the small circles along the lines). This means we look to the organization's leadership team to validate that they want us to continue to commit time and resources to furthering the development of this solution. This is an important step to take, as these points along the path are validating that the solution is **desirable, feasible**, and **viable**.

Working through each phase requires a systematic approach to answer questions, identify value, and design the right solution. We refer to these as our toolkit. A sample of these tools is available in Figure 6.4. It's important to note that different tools are used for different phases and the horizon you are looking to innovate. Using these tools will help to prepare the report that should be written at the end of each phase, which will be used to present your point of view (to move forward or end the project) to the decision-making body that releases capital (time or budget) for your projects. Whatever the decision is, this methodology captures learning and builds confidence that the right thing is being worked through the right way.

The final important piece to this puzzle is putting together the right team to work through the MVIM. Look both within and outside your organization (trusted advisors)

Frame Intent

- Commander's Intent
- Intent Statement
- Buzz Report
- Key Facts
- How Might We
- Unconference
- User Group Definition
- Market Segmentation
- Randomized Coffee Trials
- Headlines from the Future

Deep Dive

- World Café
- Semi-Structured Interview
- Ethnography
- Observation to Insights
- Ride alongs
- Compelling Experiences
- Card Sort
- Context Map
- Insight Clustering
- Journey Map
- Network Diagram
- Jobs to Be Done
- Stakeholder Map
- Personas

Generate Concepts

- Design Principles
- SCAMPER
- Worst Idea
- Precursors
- Analogs
- Business Model Canvas
- Value Proposition Canvas
- Busting Assumptions
- Scenarios
- Storyboards
- Journey Map
- Concept Cards
- Business Model Generation
- Concept Evaluation

Test

- Scenarios
- Storyboarding
- Physical Prototype
- Paper Prototype
- Digital Prototype
- Bodystorming
- MVP
- Prototype Test
- Comms Plan
- Biz Plan
- Road Map
- Capabilities IAN
- Pilot Plan

FIGURE 6.4 Saint Elizabeth Futures Toolkit

SOURCE: Copyright 2019 Saint Elizabeth Healthcare.

**Not all tools need to be completed in each phase, work through the tools until you have the confidence to present your point of view.

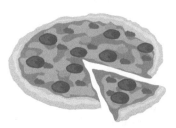

to build your team. We refer to this as the "two pizza" team. It should be no larger than the number of people who can eat two pizzas at lunch (6–8). The key is for the team to change based on what phase you are in and what expertise you need. For example, Frame Intent and Deep Dive may require subject matter experts or business and financial analysts, whereas Generate Concepts will require stakeholders, designers, product managers, and financial analysts. The Test phase will require prototypers, trainers, and project managers. Ideally, two to three individuals remain constant throughout the lifecycle.

Although at first the MVIM may seem overwhelming, working through the elements of the MVIM becomes easier with practice. In addition, not all ideas will go through the entire pipeline; in fact, the majority of them won't. Most will drop off during Frame Intent and Deep Dive as desirability, feasibility, and viability do not intersect … leaving one without the "sweet spot." If they don't, challenge yourself with the question, "Is this idea really going to have a significant impact?" Innovation in healthcare can be messy, but it's worth it when you can impact how we experience healthcare.

SUPPLEMENTAL RESOURCES

- IDEO Design Thinking
  https://designthinking.ideo.com/
- The Right Innovation Method at the Right Time
  https://hbr.org/2014/12/choose-the-right-innovation-method-at-the-right-time
- SE Health
  https://sehc.com/

Rebel Nurses at the Crossroads

PAUL KUEHNERT, DNP, RN, FAAN

"REGARDLESS OF THE SETTING, OR EVEN SECTOR, IN WHICH A NURSING JOB EXISTS, THE NURSING WORKFORCE HAS THE POTENTIAL TO HELP THE NATION REFOCUS ON HEALTH AS A HOLISTIC VALUE."

A glance at the headlines or a momentary interaction with social media can be disheartening: opioid abuse, divisive politics, and climate change. It feels as if we are living in a time of unprecedented turmoil. It is true that our 24/7 connectedness—through increasingly ubiquitous technology (on all fronts)—poses many new dilemmas. It is also true that we have weathered similar tumultuous periods in the past—periods in our history when we collectively wrung our hands and bemoaned our social ills and fractious civil discourse. Innovation is (rightfully) touted as a cure for many of these ills. I worry, however, that we nurses too often are "serial" innovators, looking for the latest and greatest solutions, rather than examining our past and asking ourselves why innovative solutions—frequently created by nurses—have failed to take hold and spread.

I look to words of wisdom from two very different American authors, William Faulkner and William Gibson, for insight on how to innovate in the face of challenging times. Faulkner said: "The past is never dead. It's not even past." And Gibson wrote: "The future is already here—it's just not evenly distributed."

The past is not even past. Nurses have long collaborated with others to create these "bright spots" that are then put forward as solutions. Think of Mary Breckenridge, who was arguably the consummate "rebel nurse." Breckenridge established the Frontier Nursing Service in 1925 to provide professional healthcare in the Appalachian Mountains of eastern Kentucky. By creating a decentralized system of nurse-midwives visiting clients in their homes, district nursing centers, and a hospital, Breckenridge and the Frontier Nursing Service lowered the maternal mortality rate in Leslie County, Kentucky, from the highest in the country to well below the national average. The key to her success? She didn't wait for permission and she didn't let conventional nursing ideologies draw artificial boundaries around her thinking. Breckenridge accomplished extraordinary things by working at the intersection of nursing and social work.

This should lead us to ask tough questions, such as why are approaches like Breckenridge's, even now, not more widespread? Have these approaches been tested in earlier/similar circumstances? Delay, when it comes to health, can literally prove fatal for the most vulnerable people we serve.

The future is already here. What are the barriers to implementation at scale? Why aren't the innovations more evenly distributed after we see positive results? I believe multiple factors limit the widespread adoption of nurse-led innovation, including inadequate allocation of resources; misalignment of payment policies; and inadequate attention to racial and class inequities in development of the models.

I came of age at the height of the Vietnam War—a time of turmoil across our nation. I cut my teeth in public health nursing at the advent of the HIV/AIDS crisis in the greater Chicago suburbs. Everything about that time felt new, too. My colleagues and I worked across professions and sectors—with social workers, faith leaders, and others—to create solutions for those suffering from a disease that had only recently gained a name and—like opioid abuse—carried a great deal of stigma. I have since realized that in helping to address the crisis in my Midwestern town, I was calling upon the skills that have been at the heart of nurses' skill set since we first became a recognized health profession: seeing and providing care to people as whole beings, whose health is shaped by their interactions with their complex, dynamic environments.

We, as nurses, have a similar and yet unique opportunity now. We know that health is greatly influenced by more than the healthcare we receive, although that's clearly important. We know that complex social and environmental factors—where we are born and live, the strength of our families and communities, the quality of our education—shape our health over our lifetimes. Wide variations in these factors mean that not everyone in our nation gets the same opportunity to experience the best possible health and well-being. Nurses have always been observers of this truth; we clearly see—often firsthand—these ills and their impact on health.

As the largest and most trusted health profession in the United States, nursing has both a unique opportunity and a corresponding responsibility to lead our nation's response. Regardless of the setting, or even sector, in which a nursing job exists, the nursing workforce has the potential to help the nation refocus on health as a holistic value. I believe we must both (as Faulkner told us) look to the past for warnings and inspiration and examine the present for trends leading toward a desired future. The "uneven distribution of the future" Gibson described creates conditions for nurses to innovate.

Innovation is so often equated with new technology; we as nurses are used to (for better or worse) working at the intersections of care and technology. Yet what about intersections of care and social conditions? While we "rebel nurses" certainly do need to seek out innovation, we need to find where the future is already present. We must think about the policy, systems, and cultural changes nurses will need to address, and what tools we'll need to give our fellow nurses in order to make these innovations work in communities across the country. How might we bring our innovative nature and holistic focus to bear on the social determinants of health?

In her 2019 report, "Activating Nursing to Address Unmet Needs in the 21st Century," Patricia Pittman, PhD, FAAN, notes that the solution lies in the original vision for our profession. She points to public health pioneer Lillian Wald, who—like Mary Breckenridge—looked beyond the boundaries set by society for her profession and addressed the social needs of her patients. "This vision," Pittman notes, "specifically at the beginning of the 20th century, and then again in the 1960s, has been grounded in a holistic focus on patients in the context of their full psychosocial well-being as members of families, workplaces, and communities" (p. 27).

Nursing stands at a crossroads: Do we work harder to establish boundaries around our profession, claiming certain services and responsibilities as only the purview of nurses? Or do we expand and diversify, as Pittman argues, welcoming "the contribution of community health workers, pharmacists, dieticians, city planners, and others, both into roles nurses have traditionally occupied, and in new spaces where nurses have been less present" (p. 29)?

The rebel nurse in me says that we should expand our horizons and soften our boundaries with others in healthcare. We should embrace working in shared and "in-between" spaces. We need to:

- Ask: Who isn't at the table who might have a part of the solution? That means looking beyond our profession—and even beyond healthcare. (Think like Walt Disney, who famously asked the overnight cleaning staff at his parks for suggestions on how to make the guest experience better.)

- Use our networks: We get so used to working in our proverbial silos that we fail to reach out to people we know who are working on similar intractable problems; people in your network will also know people you don't—and that's how innovative solutions are sustained and spread.

- Look to our pioneers: Reading the words of nurses like Lillian Wald and Mary Breckenridge remind us of tried-and-true fundamentals—fundamentals that can lay the foundation for innovation.

- Look to unusual places: While research and evidence are crucial, so is creativity. We often turn to big academia when searching for innovative solutions, yet often places with the least amount of resources are home to the most creative solutions.

By taking these steps, we will chart a new way forward for our profession, one firmly rooted in our past, but with an eye on a collective future in which everyone—regardless of circumstances—has an equal opportunity for the best possible health and well-being.

SUPPLEMENTAL RESOURCES

- Mary Breckenridge
  https://www.truthaboutnursing.org/press/pioneers/breckinridge.html
- Frontier Nursing Service
  https://frontier.edu

The Rebel Nurse's Progress Note

As you process these innovative methodologies, take note of all the practical tools provided in this publication that you can use to be an effective shift disruptor. These recommendations and concepts are not your only resources, but may serve as an initial framework of your next steps to disrupt the status quo. And, of course, at any crossroad along your rebel nurse journey, be willing and open to work between sectors and disciplines, in addition to what nursing has to offer. It is in that unique collaboration and willingness to work with others, that change is most impactful and influential. Be bold. Be ready. Be the rebel nurse who is destined to transform the future of nursing and beyond.

What other methodologies, resources, or tools have you come across recently that can continue to propel your vision to be a rebel nurse forward? Start compiling your go-to list to reference along the way.

Bibliography

Berkow, S., Virkstis, K., Stewart, J., & Conway, L. (2008). Assessing new graduate nurse performance. *Journal of Nursing Administration, 38*(11), 468–474. doi:10.1097/01.NNA.0000339477.50219.06

Clancy, C. M. (2012, January–March). Alleviating "second victim" syndrome: How we should handle patient harm. *Journal of Nursing Care Quality, 27*(1), 1–5. doi:10.1097/NCQ.0b013e3182366b53. Retrieved from http://www.ahrq.gov/news/newsroom/commentaries/second-victim-syndrome.html

Clipper, B., Wang, M., Coyne, P., Baiera, V., Love, R., Nix, D., . . . Weirich, B. (2019). *The nurse's guide to innovation: Accelerating the journey* (p. 85). Cupertino, CA: Super Star Press.

Institute of Medicine. (2000). *To err is human: Building a safer health system.* Washington, DC: National Academies Press.

Institute of Medicine. (2011). *The future of nursing: Leading change, advancing health.* Washington, DC: National Academies Press. Retrieved from http://books.nap.edu/openbook.php?record_id=12956&page=R1

ISMP. (2007, January 25). The five rights: A destination without a map. *ISMP Medication Safety Alert, 12*(2). Retrieved from http://www.ihi.org/resources/Pages/ImprovementStories/FiveRightsof MedicationAdministration.aspx

Karlöf, B., & Lövingsson, F. H. (2005). *The A–Z of management concepts and models* (pp. 209–210). London, UK: Thorogood Publishing.

Kelley, T., & Kelley, D. (2012). Reclaim your creative confidence. *Harvard Business Review.*

King, M. L., Jr. (1963). *Strength to love.* New York, NY: Harper & Row.

Knight, P. (2016). *Shoe dog: A memoir by the creator of nike* (p. 3). New York, NY: Simon and Schuster.

McKinsey Quarterly. (2009). Enduring ideas: The three horizons of growth. Retrieved from https://www.mckinsey.com/business-functions/strategy-and-corporate-finance/our-insights/enduring-ideas-the-three-horizons-of-growth

Moore, A. (2013). Tracking down Martin Luther King, Jr.'s word on health care. *Huffington Post.* Retrieved from http://www.huffingtonpost.com/amanda-moore/martin-luther-king-health-care_b_2506393.html

Orth, U. (2002). Secondary victimization of crime victims by criminal proceedings. *Social Justice Research, 15*(4), 313–325. doi:10.1023/A:1021210323461. Retrieved from https://link.springer.com/article/10.1023/A:1021210323461

Pittman, P. (2019, March 12). *Activating nursing to address unmet needs in the 21st century* (pp. 27–29). Princeton NJ: Wood Johnson Foundation.

Saint Elizabeth Healthcare. (2019). *SE Futures Toolkit. Markham,* ON, CAN: SE Futures Team.

Smith, A. (2006). *Letters to a young artist* (p. 160). New York, NY: Anchor Books.

The Chef's Garden® (2016). Chef John Folse inspires attendees at Roots 2016. Retrieved from https://www.chefs-garden.com/blog/may-2017/chef-john-folse-inspires-attendees-at-roots-2016

U.S. Food and Drug Administration (2018). Premarket notification 510(k). Retrieved from https://www.fda.gov/medical-devices/premarket-submissions/premarket-notification-510k

Walsch, N. D. (2007). *Conversations with God: An uncommon dialogue.* New York, NY: Putnam.

Wheatley, M. (2006). *Leadership and the new science: Discovering order in a chaotic world* (p. 143). San Francisco, California: Berrett-Koehler Publishers, Inc.

Williamson, M. (1992). *A return to love: Reflections on the principles of a course in miracles* (p. 192). 1st Ed. HarperCollins.

Zilm, F. (2018). The creative mind. Healthcare design: Research and theory. Retrieved from https://www.healthcaredesignmagazine.com/trends/the-creative-mind/

Appendix

PUBLICATION RESOURCES

Mary Lou Ackerman, MBA, BScN
Vice President Innovation and Digital Health
SE Health
Toronto, Ontario, Canada

- Digital Health Canada & CHIEF: Canada's Health Informatics Executive Forum. (2019). *Enterprise innovation: The current landscape of innovation in the Canadian healthcare system.* Toronto, ON, Canada: Digital Health Canada.

- Ackerman, M., Virani, T., & Billings, B. (2017). Digital mental health innovations in consumer driven care. *Nursing Leadership, 30*(3), 63–72. doi:10.12927/cjnl.2018.25384

- Ackerman, M. (2019). The promise of gerontechnology. In E. Rogers & T. Dennis (Eds.), *The future of aging* (127–189). Toronto, ON, Canada: SE Health.

Nancy M. Albert, PhD, CCNS, CHFN, CCRN, NE-BC, FAHA, FCCM, FHFSA, FAAN
Associate Chief Nursing Officer, Research and Innovation-Nursing Institute and Clinical Nurse Specialist, Heart Failure-Kaufman Center for Heart failure in the Heart and Vascular Institute
Cleveland Clinic
Cleveland, Ohio

- Albert, N. M. (Ed.). (2016). *Building and sustaining a hospital-based nursing research program.* New York, NY: Springer Publishing Company.

- Handberg, E., Albert, N. M., Clark, A. P., Feeley-Coe, P., Cooper, J., Gorski, K. A., . . . Zarling, K. K. (Task Force Members). (2008). *Cardiovascular nursing: Scope and standards of practice.* Silver Spring, MD: Nursebooks.org (American Nurses Association).

Shawna Butler, DNP, JD, RN, CPHRM
Patient Safety Specialist/Research Nurse Coordinator/Nurse, Massachusetts General Hospital, Boston, Massachusetts
Nursing Faculty, University of Massachusetts, Boston, Massachusetts

- Butler, S.M. (2020). Adverse Events, in Gross, K.A. (Ed.) *Advanced practice and leadership in radiology nursing* (p. 213–221). Cham, Switzerland: Springer Nature.

BONNIE CLIPPER, DNP, RN, MA, MBA, CENP, FACHE
CHIEF CLINICAL OFFICER
WAMBI
AUSTIN, TEXAS

- Clipper, B., Wang, M., Coyne, P., Baiera, V., Love, R., Nix, D., ... Weirich, B. (2019). *The nurse's guide to innovation.* Cupertino, CA: Super Star Press.

- Clipper, B. (2012). *The nurse manager's guide to an intergenerational workforce.* Indianapolis, IN: Sigma Theta Tau Publishing.

PAUL E. COYNE, DNP, MBA, MS, RN, APRN, AGPCNP-BC
PRESIDENT AND CO-FOUNDER
INSPIREN
ASSISTANT VICE PRESIDENT, CLINICAL PRACTICE & CHIEF NURSING INFORMATICS OFFICER
HOSPITAL FOR SPECIAL SURGERY
NEW YORK, NEW YORK

- Clipper, B., Wang, M., Coyne, P., Baiera, V., Love, R., Nix, D., ... Weirich, B. (2019). *The nurses guide to innovation.* Cupertino, CA: Super Star Press.

MARGARET A. FITZGERALD, DNP, FNP-BC, NP-C, FAANP, CSP, FAAN, DCC, FNAP
FOUNDER, FITZGERALD HEALTH EDUCATION ASSOCIATES
CLINICAL PRACTICE, FAMILY NURSE PRACTITIONER, GREATER LAWRENCE (MA) FAMILY
  HEALTH CENTER
ADJUNCT ASSOCIATE PROFESSOR, FRANCES PAYNE BOLTON SCHOOL OF NURSING, CASE
  WESTERN RESERVE UNIVERSITY, CLEVELAND, OHIO

- Fitzgerald, M. A. (2020). *Nurse practitioner certification examination and practice preparation* (6th ed.). Philadelphia, PA: F. A. Davis.

JOAN GURVIS SHIELDS, MSN, RN, BCC
SENIOR FACULTY/LEADERSHIP SOLUTIONS PARTNER
CENTER FOR CREATIVE LEADERSHIP
COLORADO SPRINGS, COLORADO

- Van Velsor, E., & Gurvis, J. (2007). Experiential learning in leadership development. In M. Silberman (Ed.), *The handbook of experiential learning* (pp. 306–320). San Francisco, CA: Pfeiffer.

- Calarco, A., & Gurvis, J. (2005). *Adaptability: Responding effectively to change. CCL ideas into action guidebook for the practicing manager.* Colorado Springs, CO: CCL Press.

- Editorial Board. (2000). *Health care curriculum resource manual.* Gaithersburg, MD: Aspen Publications.

- Gurvis, J., Ouimette, R., & Friedman, B. (1996). Preceptorship in primary care. In J. Hickey, R. Ouimette, & S. Venegon (Eds.), *Advanced practice nursing: Changing roles and clinical applications* (pp. 54–62). Philadelphia, PA: J. B. Lippincott.

- Gurvis, J. (1992). Gestational diabetes. In G. Stamps & L. G. Vonfrolio (Eds.), *Nursing review book: Maternal child health.* Springhouse, PA: Springhouse.

Paul Kuehnert, DNP, RN, FAAN
Associate Vice President-Program, Robert Wood Johnson Foundation, Princeton, New Jersey
Affiliate Professor of Nursing, University of Washington, Seattle, Washington

- Leviton, L., Kuehnert, P., & Wehr, K. (2019). Public health: A transformation in the 21st century. In J. Knickman & B. Elbel (Eds.), *Jonas and Kovner's health care delivery in the United States* (12th ed., pp. 123–150). New York, NY: Springer Publishing Company.

- Kuehnert, P. L. (2017). Ending business as usual: The Kane County health department in a worsening fiscal limate. *Journal of Public Health Management and Practice, 23(2)*, 178–186.

- Kuehnert, P., & Plough, A. (2017). Improving population health. In R. Bialek, L. Beitsch, J. Moran (Eds.), *Solving population health problems through collaboration*. Boca Raton, FL: Taylor & Francis.

- Kuehnert, P. L. (2018). Overview of program planning. In N. E. Ervin & P. Kulbok (Ed.), *Advanced community health nursing practice: Population-focused care* (2nd ed., pp. 203–220). New York, NY: Springer Publishing Company.

- Kuehnert, P. L., Matthes, T., & White, W. L. (1998). A cooperative model of HIV case management: Evaluation and research issues from Chicago. *Evaluating HIV Case Management: Invited Research & Evaluation Papers. Health Resources and Services Administration, HIV/AIDS Bureau,* 146–160.

- Figert, A., & Kuehnert, P. L. (1997). Reframing knowledge about the AIDS epidemic: Academic and community-based interventions. In P. Nyden, A. Figert, M. Shibley, & D. Burrows (Eds.), *Building community: Social science in action* (pp. 154–160). Thousand Oaks, CA: Pine Forge Press.

Nicole Lincoln, MS, RN, FNP-BC, CCNS, CCRN
Senior Manager of Nursing Innovations
Boston Medical Center
Boston, Massachusetts

- Lewis, K., Canelli, R., & Ortega, R. (2018). *OK to proceed? What every health care provider should know about patient safety.* Boston, MA: Boston Medical Center. Retrieved from https:oktoproceed.com

Amy Rose Taylor, AGNP-BC, BSN, RN
Clinical Services Manager
Optum at Home, UnitedHealth Group
Pennsylvania

- Taylor, A. R. (2015). *Nursing School 101: How to get into, through, and out of nursing school and into a job you will love.* Washington, DC: Difference Press

Debbie Toomey, RN, CIPP
Speaker–Author–Consultant
Founder, President
Ultimate Healing Journey, LLC
Quincy, Massachusetts

- Toomey, D. L. (2014). December 26, in E. Harper & C. Connor (Eds.), *365 days of angel prayers* (p. 434). North Charleston, SC: Create Space.
- Toomey, D. L. (2016). *The happiness result—More time, more health, more love, more success. 7 simple techniques to create your A.W.E.S.O.M.E.™ life.* Quincy, MA: Borromeo Publishing.
- Toomey, D. L. (2016). *The happiness result—Goals, gratitude, & success journal. For manifesting goals, giving thanks, and celebrating success along the way.* Quincy, MA: Borromeo Publishing.
- Toomey, D. L. (2017). *The happiness result—Art therapy coloring book. Express & enjoy tourself.* Quincy, MA: Borromeo Publishing

JENNIFER WALLACE, MSN, RN
ASSISTANT PROFESSOR
FAMILY FOCUSED NURSING
LAWRENCE MEMORIAL REGIS COLLEGE
MEDFORD, MASSACHUSETTS

- Wallace, J., & Ridpath-Parker, J. (1993). Kangaroo care. *Quality Management in Health Care, 2*(1), 1–5. doi:10.1097/00019514-199300000-00004
- Curley, M., & Wallace, J. (1992). Effects of the nursing Mutual Participation Model of Care in the pediatric intensive care unit—a replication. *Journal of Pediatric Nursing, 7*(6), 377–385.
- Johnson, B. H., Jeppson, E. S., & Redburn, L. (1992). *Caring for children and families: Guidelines for hospitals.* Bethesda, MD: Association for the Care of Children's Health.

KEVIN WHITNEY, DNP, RN, NEA-BC
SENIOR VICE PRESIDENT OF PATIENT CARE SERVICES & CHIEF NURSING OFFICER
NEWTON-WELLESLEY HOSPITAL
NEWTON, MASSACHUSETTS

- Whitney, K., Haag-Heitman, B., Chisholm, M., & Gale, S. (2018). Nursing peer review perceptions and practices. In S. Ahmed, L. Andrist, S. Davis, & V. Fuller (Eds.), *DNP education, practice, and policy; Mastering the DNP essentials for advanced nursing practice* (2nd ed., p. 171). New York, NY: Springer Publishing Company.
- Whitney, K., Burke, D., Gallivan, T., & Tenney, D. (2013). Designing the infrastructure to foster nurse-led care at the bedside. In J. Ives-Erickson, D. A. Jones, & M. Ditomassi (Eds.), *Fostering nurse-led care: Professional practice for the bedside leader from Massachusetts General Hospital* (pp. 241–258). Indianapolis, IN: Sigma Theta Tau International.

WENDY WRIGHT, DNP, ANP-BC, FNP-BC, FAANP, FAAN, FNAP
ADULT AND FAMILY NURSE PRACTITIONER
OWNER, WRIGHT & ASSOCIATES FAMILY HEALTHCARE @ AMHERST AND @ CONCORD, NEW HAMPSHIRE
ADJUNCT FACULTY, FAY W. WHITNEY SCHOOL OF NURSING, UNIVERSITY OF WYOMING, LARAMIE, WYOMING

- Wright, W. L. (2017). *Adult physical assessment cue cards* (9th ed.). Andover, MA: Fitzgerald Health Education Associates.

Index